Let's Talk Back

Second Edition

By

Barbara Simon

First Edition Sold Out In 2 Weeks!

EDES PUBLISHING CO.

Let's Talk Back

By Barbara Simon

www.backcaresolutions.net

ISBN-13: 978-0-9788010-4-5
ISBN-10: 0-9788010-4-0

Made in the United States of America

Dedication

Some words of thanks to my always supportive husband who went through the process of developing this book with me and had to endure hours of proof reading, discussions about grammar and taking pictures. He definitely knows Dorn Spinal Therapy inside out now hence he has a very healthy back. And in case that changes he knows exactly what he has to do.

I also would like to thank my children Luca and Leoni who never have given up on me and believed in the fact that this book would be available to the public one day. Their trust led me through a few hiccups and wanting to give up, but I didn't want to disappoint them – and in the end of course myself.

So thank you my dear family, you are the best I have.

Barbara/Mum

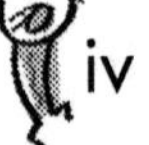

Foreword

Dear Reader,

I am proud to present this valuable little book to you and hope that you will benefit from reading it and doing the exercises within it.

A few years ago when I started working as a Dorn Spinal therapist in Germany, I never would have thought that one day I would be living in Sydney. I perform and teach Dorn Spinal Therapy here, to help many people overcome their back or neck pain. Now, I'm writing this book with exercises that people all over the world can access and use to become active in eliminating their back pain.

Life is full of surprises and no-one knows what is written in their diary of life. Therefore, it is good to be prepared, and keep your body and mind in shape. You then can take on all the surprises that await you, with an open mind and a healthy body.

Don't miss out on what could potentially be the biggest events in your life just because you don't feel well! Don't let pain or lack of fitness, mental and/or physical, come your way. Act

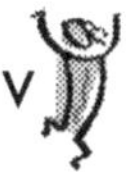

early enough before it becomes chronic. If you already suffer from a chronic disease, don't give up. There is always hope. Keep an open mind, and you will find a solution for your problem – maybe it is Dorn Spinal Therapy.

I wish you all the best and trust that you will be successful using this book and getting to know your first Dorn therapist.

Barbara Simon
Sydney, Australia –September 2007

Disclaimer:

Before you start reading this book I must express the importance of seeking medical attention when you have strong pain or after you have had an accident, a fall, or injured your back in any other circumstances. It is important to rule out any fractures, ruptures or other conditions that may be detrimental to proceeding with any of the exercises contained in this book. These exercises are good to add to your already existing exercises or start up your own routine to keep your back healthy. If you are not sure about how to do certain exercises, seek advice from a Dorn Spinal therapist or, if no local therapist, from your doctor or health practitioner or physiotherapist.

Here's the fine print:

The information contained in this book is educational in nature. The author has made every effort to ensure that all information is complete and accurate. However, the information and advice contained in this book is not intended as a substitute for consulting your doctor or health practitioner regarding any action that may affect your well- being. Individual readers must assume responsibility for their own actions, safety and health. The author shall not be liable or responsible for any loss, injury or damage what-so-ever allegedly arising from any information, exercise or other suggestion contained in this book.

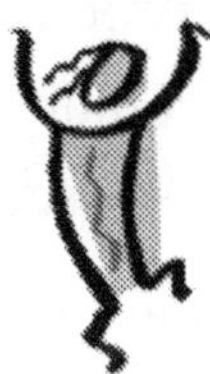

Table of Contents

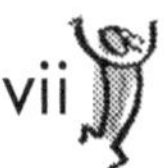

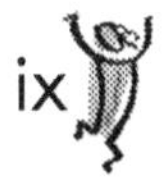

Introduction

Healing with special touches and movements of the spine and joints dates back to the origin of modern humans. The manual therapy of Dorn also goes back to folk medicine. The experiences of different healers over the years have been brought together to form a complete therapy. This offers a new possibility for anyone suffering from any sort of back pain, neck pain and/or headaches.

Not only does it offer a new treatment approach for practitioners, it also has a wide range of self-help exercises that enable you to speed up your own healing process and make you more independent from practitioners.

In Part One of this book I will explain the main common facts of back pain and the basic knowledge about the pain related to body parts and functions. Please do yourself a favour and read this information carefully. It is vital to understand the different causes of pain as well as the basics of your spine, especially if you intend to work on it by yourself.

I will then introduce the basics of the Dorn Spinal Therapy. Furthermore, I will explain the differences between the most popular and competing treatment, Chiropractic, and why the Dorn Spinal Therapy, in particular, is an ideal self-help for back pain-related problems.

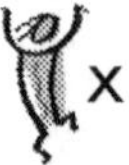

Part Two of the book contains the exercises to relieve your back and neck pain by yourself in the most simple but efficient way, anytime and anywhere! You can refer to that section whenever you need a "quick fix."

Part Three will give you some vital information about the do's and don'ts for a better back as well as some additional self-help modalities.

Last but not least I would like to stress that all your comments on this self-help guide are highly welcome. Whenever you have a question or a suggestion for an improvement just send an e-mail to info@backcaresolutions.net Of course I would love to hear success stories: how you beat your back pain and how this book has made a difference to your wellbeing in dealing with one of the most common medical problems in our modern society.

One more thing:
Back Care Solutions always tries to provide you with the latest and most helpful information possible. But at the end of the day it is YOU who has to put them in place. I am confident that if you take action, and do the exercises on a regular basis **you will succeed**. Do your body a big favour by looking after yourself and you will be rewarded for it in the long term. Your journey to a pain-free back can start here and now. I know that Dorn Spinal Therapy is a very effective treatment and not only do I practice and teach it, I am confident that

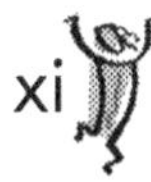

in no time there will be more practitioners in Australia and around the world. The growing interest in this therapy will afford a chance for everyone to experience the treatment and the benefits. So keep on asking for Dorn Spinal therapists in your area and help make this technique more popular.

I am running training courses for interested people, not only therapists but anyone who would like to help family and/or friends with their back pain. It is an easy-to-learn technique and you do not need much knowledge of anatomy and physiology. For more information go to www.backcaresolutions.net and click on the workshop link.

I hope you enjoy reading this book and learning how to help yourself with your pain management, and of course recommending it to other people with back and/or neck pain.

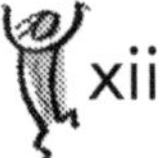

1

THE DORN SPINAL THERAPY

1.1 The Spine

1.1.1 The Vertebrae

Main Parts

- the spinous processes (the bony ends we can feel on the spine)
- 2 transverse processes, one on each side
- the vertebral foramen, where the bone marrow sits
- the vertebral body

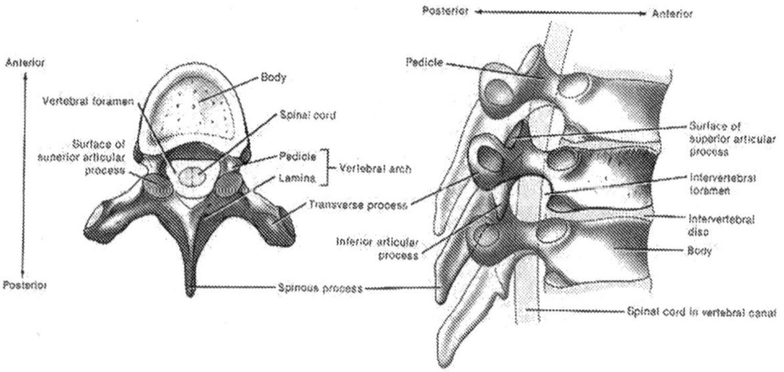

The spine is nowhere near as fragile as we might think, therefore it is not a problem to work on it with a fair amount of pressure, given no osteoporosis is evident.

The vertebrae are connected by cartilage and joints and are secured by lots of different ligaments.

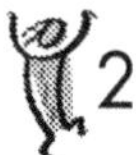

1.1.2 The Discs

In-between the vertebrae there are the discs. They consist of fibrous cartilage and inside have an aqueous nucleus pulposus, a little ball-like water cushion.

The discs make sure we are flexible when we bend and with this action the nucleus shifts. When we experience a prolapsed disc, that is when the nucleus has been pressed out of the disc (see picture) and is in contact with the nerve, producing various degrees of pain.

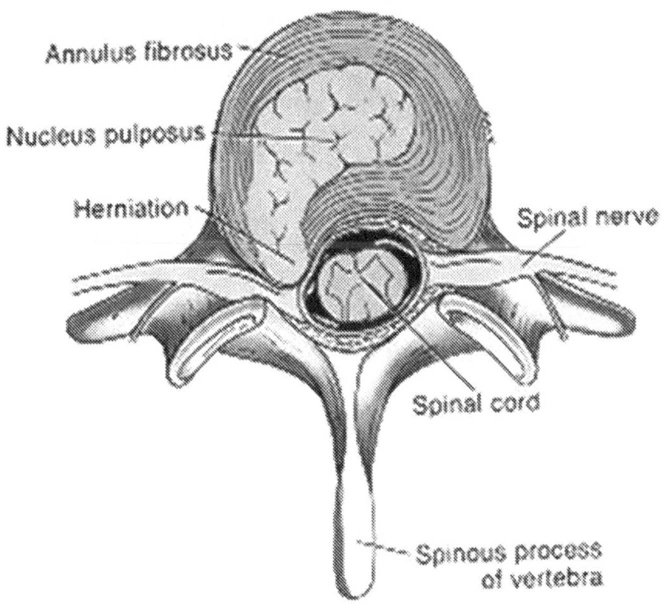

The spine keeps the head upright, carries the skull and supports the shoulders and pelvic girdle.

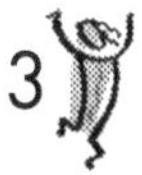

The vertebral body becomes bigger, the further down we look, so as to carry more weight.

The shape of the spine is a double "S" which helps protect the very sensitive brain from vibration and withstands the impact which walking, jumping, sports, etc., have on our spine. It also ensures elasticity and flexibility of the spine.

Looking at the vertebrae from the top down, the vertebral foramen form the vertebral canal in which we find the marrow. In between the vertebrae we find a hole, the intervertebral foramen, through which the spinal nerves emerge. Those spinal nerves play a crucial part in the support and nourishment of our body's organs and functions.

The human being is the only vertebrate with a bend between lumbar vertebrae and sacrum, due to walking upright. We obviously pay a high price for being upright as problems in the area of lumbar vertebra 3-5 are much more common than in any other areas.

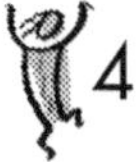

1.1.3 Reasons For Abnormally Positioned Vertebrae

Often when patients ask the reason for their pain they are told that their discs have worn down. That can be a little bit misleading. Every cell of the body rejuvenates itself permanently and that happens also in the spine and the discs.

In other words, if our body parts were to wear down, the first ones would be our hands and fingers, but they remain the same length, regardless of whether you use your hands for gentle or hard work. Regarding the discs in the spine, it would be more precise to speak of deformations rather than of wearing down. On the other hand there are cases where discs or vertebrae can be damaged faster than the body is able to replace the damaged parts – especially the older the patient gets.

Why Discs "Slip"

- upright walking
- lack of movement
- diet
- shock
- stress
- accident
- prenatal scoliosis
- leg length difference
- weak muscles
- emotional problems

The abnormal positions of the discs due to various deformations are numerous.

The main reason is walking upright, the second main cause is the lack of movement and exercise. Prenatal scoliosis, shock and stress, accidents, high strain e.g. right or left handedness, differences in leg length and many more circumstances can lead to a "slipped" disc.

The muscles are also part of pain experiences. In particular, the deeper lying back Erector is a pain source. Neck pain often results from a stiff Trapezius muscle. Stress and wrong posture lead to tightening of smaller muscle groups between the vertebrae and the superficial transverse muscles.

It is good to loosen the tight muscles through specific exercises, massage, hot baths with Epsom Salts, etc. on a regular basis. Just as you take your car to regular services for maintenance, your body deserves the same attention. This way it should last you longer than any car you will have in your life. So don't you think your body deserves more attention?

To reduce the pressure on the discs you have to make sure you strengthen **all** the muscles: leg, arm, and, extremely important, the tummy and back muscles.

A common reason for tight muscles is wrong diet. The organism is acidic, we eat too much salt, drink too much cof-

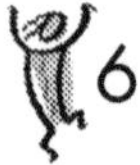

fee, and we don't drink enough water. Also emotional problems like anxiety, anger, grief or a very rigid attitude can be responsible for tight muscles which can change the whole body posture.

If the affected person finds no way to adequately solve the problems he/she is facing, these tight muscles become tighter and shorter, leading to pain in the neck and shoulder area as well as in the rest of the back. This pain then stresses the person and the emotional burden leads to even worse posture, resulting in a vicious cycle.

It is important to distinguish if this is a person's inner attitude or if they are taking on the attitude of another person like a relative, friend, colleague or employer. Realising these connections is a big task when working with people suffering from back pain. Final resolutions with these issues, though, is always the person's own responsibility.

Louise L. Hay, author of many healing books, says: "all disease comes out of non-forgiveness". She divides a person's back into 3 parts, upper, middle and lower back and draws conclusions in regards to the pain:

- upper back pain – person doesn't feel enough emotional support
- middle back pain– person could be dealing with guilt, anxiety, fear to face some hidden issues

- lower back pain – financial concerns.

Hay's suggestion for solving these problems is to train new mind-settings and train them until the inner and outer attitude conform. A good exercise to start with new mind-settings is to tell yourself in front of a mirror every day as often as possible:

- for general back pain: *I know that life always supports me*
- for upper back pain: *I love and accept myself. Life loves and supports me.*
- for middle back pain: *I let go of the past. I am free to move forward with a loving heart.*
- for lower back pain: *I trust the process of life. Everything I need has been taken care of. I am safe.*

I do not say, that these affirmations - or affirmations in general - will heal your back problems once and for all. But positive attitude training has helped and supported many people on their way to achieve better health.

With these affirmations, which everyone can take on board, you also take responsibility back into your own life. A therapist can only lead the way and offer their help. The patient must start walking **alone** as healing lies only **within.**

Many people feel fear about expressing the reality of their

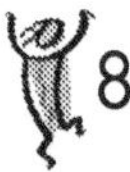

situations and how they feel about them. The pressure, socially, in family affairs as well as work related, is increasing constantly and it is getting more and more difficult to do what we, as individuals, really need.

For example someone might say: “I have to work too much” but in reality feels and means: “I am not getting enough recognition and support“. Or you might say: “I have stress” but really mean that you take too little time out for relaxation and resting. If you feel your situation puts a heavy strain on you, you may need someone to help you share the burden. Then it is up to you to ask for the help you need and you will get it if you persist.

A lot of emotional conditions can lead to some sort of back pain but if you realise it, it is up to you to change it and bring healing into your life.

Unfortunately most people do not listen to their body so instead of taking time off to get professional help, they would rather take medication, hoping to find relief. But the pain does not go away and after some time the pain leads to postural changes and even to stiffening. Flexibility is reduced and the next step is sprains, pulled muscles, torn ligaments. Here it is again – the vicious cycle.

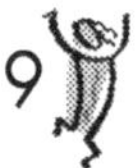

1.1.4 Consequences Of An Unaligned Spine

Even the smallest slipping or tilting of a disc in the spine can cause damage of the nerve, best known for example with sciatic pain, due to the nerves originating in the spine. For sciatica it is normally the nerves between the 4th and 5th lumbar spine or from the different vertebral foramen of the sacrum.

In the upper back you can experience pain similar to "lumbago" if a vertebra becomes tilted and squeezes the nerve due to an unfortunate movement. The immediate pain is the consequence of a so-called myogelosis, hardened muscles that hold the slipped vertebrae in the required position to avoid worse things happening.

While the vertebra remains uncorrected, the pain will stay and cause more muscles to harden. So the best advice in this case is to see a Dorn Spinal therapist as soon as possible and use a heat pack or hot water bottle to reduce the stiffening of the muscles.

The majority of spinal problems though may not be as immediately noticeable. They can remain unnoticed for a long time. Therefore people often don't understand why they suffer from back pain all of a sudden without having done any-

thing "wrong" or having had any kind of accident.

In other cases they might suffer from organ problems and the doctor treats those, without real success, whereas the real cause is in the spine: the nerve that has been trapped, went numb and stopped the support of the related organ.

Whenever you experience organ problems, like recurring bladder infections, kidney stones, digestive problems, headaches, asthma, even allergies and you can't find any relief it is definitely worthwhile having a Dorn Spinal Therapy treatment done to make sure the spine is straight and not the cause of the problems.

1.1.5 Possible Aches and Pains Due To Wrongly Positioned Vertebrae

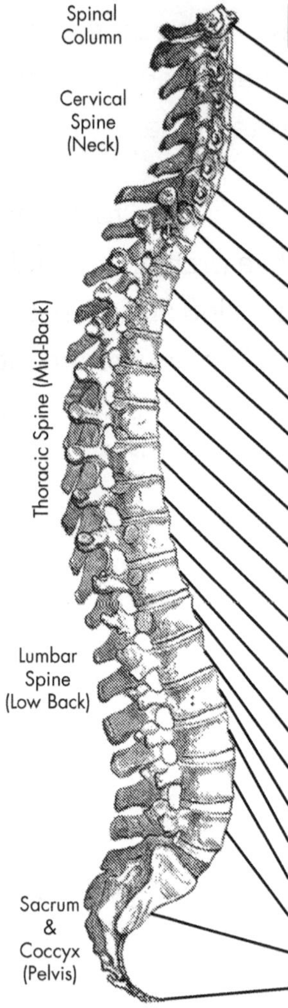

Spinal Column
Cervical Spine (Neck)
Thoracic Spine (Mid-Back)
Lumbar Spine (Low Back)
Sacrum & Coccyx (Pelvis)

Vertebrae	Areas & Parts of Body
1C	Back at the head
2C	Various areas of the head
3C	Side and front of the neck
4C	Upper back of neck
5C	Middle of neck and upper part of arms
6C	Lower pan of neck, arms, and elbows
7C	Lower part of arms, shoulders
1T	Fiends: wrists, fingers, thyroid
2T	Heart, its valves and coronary arteries
3T	Lungs, bronchial tubes. pleura, chest
4T	Gall bladder. common duct
5T	Liver. solar plexus
6T	Stomach, mid-back area
7T	Pancreas, duodenum
8T	Spleen, lower mid-back
9T	Adrenal glands
10T	Kidneys
11T	Ureters
12T	Small intestines, upperlower back
1L	Iliocecal valve, large intestines
2L	Appendix, abdomen, upper leg
3L	Sex organs, uterus, bladder, knees
4L	Prostate gland, lower back
5L	Sciatic nerve, lower legs, ankles, feet
Sacrum	Hip bones. buttocks
Coccyx	Rectum, anus

Cervical Vertebra 1 = Atlas:

<u>Physical problems:</u>

Headaches, high blood pressure, migraines, amnesia, fatigue, vertigo, partial paralysis due to uneven circulation of brain halves

Emotional problems:

Lack of overview, missing connection to higher self, wanting to deal with things intellectually only, not trusting their spirit

Cervical Vertebra 2 = Axis

Physical problems:

Sinusitis, eye problems, deafness, ear aches

Emotional problems:

Missing “vision“, not wanting to look at problems closely

Cervical Vertebra 3

Physical problems:

Facial nerve pain, pimples, acne, tinnitus, tooth-ache, neuralgia

Emotional problems:

Not wanting to listen, not having a strong stance, very volatile, feelings of guilt

Cervical Vertebra 4

Physical problems:

Permanent sneezing, loss of hearing, polyps, catarrh

Emotional problems:

See Cervical Vertebra 3

Cervical Vertebra 5

Physical problems:

Hoarseness, sore throat, chronic colds, laryngitis

Emotional problems:

Unable to talk well, feel as if there is a lump in the throat

Cervical Vertebra 6

Physical problems:

Tonsillitis, croup, stiff neck, upper arm pain, whooping cough, goitre

Emotional problems:

See Cervical Vertebra 5

Cervical Vertebra 7

Physical problems:

Thyroid problems, colds, bursitis in shoulders, depression, anxiety

Emotional problems:

Feel suppressed, suffer quietly, unable to stand up for self

Thoracic Vertebrae 1

Physical problems:
Shoulder pain, stiffening neck, pain in lower arm and hand, tendonitis, tennis arm, numbness in fingers
Emotional problems:
Carry a lot on their shoulders, do everything on their own, no trust

Thoracic Vertebrae 2

Physical problems:
Heart problems, anxiety, pain in the chest
Emotional problems:
Cannot be deeply loving, closed heart, lack of joy

Thoracic Vertebrae 3

Physical problems:
Bronchitis, flu, pneumonia, cough, breathing problems, asthma
Emotional problems:
Putting oneself in the background, unable to breathe through, no personal opinion or the complete opposite: greedy, egotistic, unable to share

Thoracic Vertebrae 4

Physical problems:
Gallbladder problems, gallstones, hepatitis, lateral headache
Emotional problems:
Inner anger, keeping all to self, feeling of bitterness, hard on self, overly focused

Thoracic Vertebrae 5

Physical problems:
Liver problems, low blood pressure, anaemia, fatigue, shingles, weak circulatory system, arthritis
Emotional problems:
Worry about others, problems with the "inner child", unable to look after their own interests, often sad, cry a lot

Thoracic Vertebrae 6

Physical problems:
Stomach problems, digestive problems, heartburn, diabetes, pancreatic problems
Emotional problems:
Choke a lot, unable to release things, internally rebellious, lost in addictions

Thoracic Vertebrae 7

Physical problems:

Duodenal ulcers, stomach problems, hiccups

Emotional problems:

See Thoracic Vertebra 6

Thoracic Vertebrae 8

Physical problems:

Spleen problems, weak immunity

Emotional problems:

Worry a lot, suppress “flow of life“

Thoracic Vertebrae 9

Physical problems:

Allergies, urticaria

Emotional problems:

Suppress own aggressions, develop allergies, make reproaches

Thoracic Vertebrae 10

Physical problems:

Kidney problems, arteriosclerosis, fatigue

Emotional problems:

Problems in social relationship with parents, partners, children, colleagues etc.

Thoracic Vertebrae 11

Physical problems:

Acne, pimples, eczema, psoriasis

Emotional problems:

Problems with making contacts, insecurity, always seeing own weaknesses, anxious

Thoracic Vertebrae 12

Physical problems:

Bloating, rheumatitis, growth disturbance, infertility

Emotional problems:

New beginnings are difficult, can't release past, anxious\

Lumbar Vertebrae 1

Physical problems:

Imbalances in the large intestines, colonial bleedings, constipation, diarrhoea

Emotional problems:

See Thoracic Vertebra 12

Lumbar Vertebrae 2

Physical problems:

Appendicitis, stomach cramps, acidosis, varicose veins

Emotional problems:

Tighten up easily, feelings of panic

Lumbar Vertebrae 3

Physical problems:

Problems during pregnancy, PMT, problems with menopause, bladder problems, knee pain, impotence, bed wetting

Emotional problems:

Sexual problems, slow in "digesting" things, lacking warmth and security

Lumbar Vertebrae 4

Physical problems:

Sciatica, prostate problems, painful or frequent urinating

Emotional problems:

See Lumbar Vertebra 3

Lumbar Vertebrae 5

Physical problems:

Circulation problems of the lower limbs and feet, cold feet, calf cramps, swelling of feet and legs

Emotional problems:

See Lumbar Vertebra 3

Sacrum

Physical problems:

Sciatica, pelvic problems, chronic constipation, pain in feet and legs

Emotional problems:

Overburdened by life, Inactivity

Coccyx

Physical problems:

Haemorrhoids, rectal itching, pain sitting down

Emotional problems:

Out of balance with yourself. Holding on. Blame of self. Sitting on old pain.

These are only a few possibilities regarding problems that can arise due to an unaligned spine.

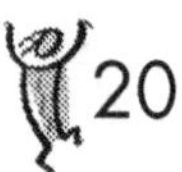

Generally speaking it is always worth a visit with a Dorn Spinal therapist if you experience any sort of physical problem that can't be solved in another therapeutic way. As a complementary form of treating the emotional problems it is worth taking a look at Bach Flower or Bush Flower essences as they offer a very gentle way of helping you address your emotional problems.

1.2 Principals And Fundamentals Of The Dorn Spinal Therapy

The Dorn Spinal Therapy is not only a spinal and joint therapy, but also a whole body therapy as we work close to the spine and therefore also on the nerves.

- Correcting the Joints - joints out of place can lead to joint cavity which means a blockage in the energy flow and, after some time, resulting pain.

- Holistic Treatment - all joints in the lower limbs, the pelvis and the whole spine to be checked as symptoms in completely different body areas can still be related to problems in the spine. For example a blocked 2nd cervical vertebra can cause constant ear ache, visual problems or sinusitis.

- Movement - a fundamental element in the treatment. All corrections happen in dynamics, the patient is swinging either his leg, arm or moving his head, depending on the area the therapist is working on. The movement "distracts" the muscles which makes the correction easier. This speciality makes the treatment a gentle therapy.

- Pain Threshold - the Dorn Spinal therapist never goes

beyond it. Pain can't be avoided completely, but as soon as it is too much the therapist stops working on that particular part. The work then continues at a later time.

- Low Repetition Treatments - the average amount of treatments needed is 3-4, depending how chronic the problem is.

- Prevention - a vital part of the Dorn Spinal Therapy as necessary corrections can be undertaken before they cause any pain and bigger problems. Therefore it is advised to have a preventative treatment once every 6-12 months, after all it is also a very relaxing treatment which can be enjoyed by everyone.

- Check-ups - ideal for babies, children and young adults as it is a non-invasive and simple technique to prevent or cure misalignments in earlier ages.

1.2.1 Why Do Joints Slip Out Of Their Ideal Position?

Joint	Behaviour
Hip joint	• deep sitting, for example in a soft lounge or car seat • sitting with crossed legs • bending over with straight knees • certain stretching exercises • falls or strong pushes
Knee joint	• improper strain • bending for more than 90° • sitting on the heels • certain stretch and/or twisting exercises • falls or strong pushes
Ankle joint	• going over the ankle • twisting of feet around chair legs • certain stretches • falls or strong pushes

1.2.2 Early Signs And Long-Term Consequences Of An Uneven Pelvis

- You cannot stand on both legs at the same time over a long period of time
- You shift from one leg to another or seem to be swaying
- Back pain in the lower back or groin area and/or hip pain
- Pain while lying down
- Knee pain

Middle or long-term, the one-sided strain can lead to serious negative effects such as:

- Hip degenerative joint disease
- Severe sciatic pain in the shorter leg
- Tensions in the shoulder girdle
- Positional changes of one or more vertebrae along the spine
- Jaw joint problems
- Problems in the reproductive system or digestive system
- Foot problems, etc.

You may never have thought about the weight that is on your vertebrae and discs every time you carry a child, a heavy basket, shopping bags or even the position in which you sit. But this pressure stresses your spine every day, compresses your discs more and more and can cause a difference in your height of up to 5 cm. That is why we are shorter at night. Only by regenerating during the night can the discs expand, increasing the distance between the vertebrae, and hopefully - the spine will work properly the next day and the next and the next.

Now imagine having just 1 or 2 slipped or tilted vertebrae or discs in your spine and the problems this can create. The fact is that the aging process in the body starts at about 20 years of age and the discs are affected from then on. The nucleus loses liquid and therefore the protective capacity is reduced over the years.

Although every single cell in the body regenerates over and over again, the process slows down the older we get. At some stage even a restful night's sleep does not lead to a complete regeneration anymore.

If, on top of that, there are also some abnormal positions of vertebrae or postural problems, subsequent back and neck pain is inevitable - at some stage even a prolapsed disc.
The duty of a Dorn Spinal therapist therefore, is first of all to check the joints and vertebrae for any blockages and abnor-

mal positions. As soon as something has been found, the corrective handling, in a gentle but decisive way and with the help of the client, takes place. Only when all joints are corrected, the structure is right and the energy flow is open, aches, pains and/or reduced movements can slowly start to heal.

1.2.3 How Does A Dorn Spinal Therapist Work?

The only prerequisite for a treatment is that the person seeking help is still able to move and stand genuinely. Generally speaking the treatment causes no or light pain but a responsible therapist never works beyond the pain threshold of a patient.

After the treatment one can experience up to four days of sore muscle pain due to the shifting of musculo-skeletal systems in the body. Stretching exercises and physical exertion should be avoided for about a week so that the tissue, ligaments and tendons have time to adjust themselves and support the system again.

It is very important that the patient drinks **a lot** of water - two to three litres a day minimum. The toxins that are released with the treatment have to be flushed out of the body so they can not cause other damage in the system.

The first thing a Dorn Spinal therapist does is check your leg length. About 85% of people have a difference in leg length, often without knowing. These differences can vary between 1mm and 5cm!

Many people, who are aware of it, have a built-up heel under the shoe or a heel support in the shoe. Unfortunately mostly under the healthy leg (the shorter leg), as the longer leg is the "pathological" one.

Experience has shown that most differences are due to incorrectly fitted joints. Among these, the hip joint is the most common one. By actually measuring the legs themselves you would find any differences that indicate a structural problem. The therapist uses a simple exercise to get the "longer" leg back into the right position in the joint, which means making the longer leg shorter not vice-versa as most other modalities do. The client maintains that position with easy exercises, which are shown later on.

While the most common incorrect joint is the hip joint, we also find problems in knee and/or ankle joints and the sacrum. A subluxation in this area can create all sorts of problems.

Most hips need about three to four alignments. After each alignment the therapist measures the legs again until they are completely balanced and straight. In some cases both legs seem to be even but starting the checking process and adjustment actually might show that on both sides there are subluxations in the joints that end up with the same difference on both sides. So therefore it is very important to really check the legs, even if they appear to be the same length.

The next step in a Dorn treatment is the balancing of the pelvis.

In most cases of different leg lengths there is also a twisted hip due to the fact that the longer leg pushes the hip slightly up and/or forward or back. This imbalance is corrected in movement with the client and then we can move on to the spine itself to check for deviations in the spine.

Most times the deviation area is sore when pushing on it, which is another indicator that something is not quite right in that area. Working here requires the cooperation of the client and once finished with the whole spine we then move on to the Spinal Stretch Massage to relax and nurture the spine and the back itself.

1.2.4 Comparison Of Chiropractic And Dorn Therapy Treatments

The Dorn Spinal Therapy is different from any type of spinal treatment and the only factor in common with Chiropractic is that they both work on the spine and joints.

With chiropractic, the corrections are done with the patient at rest and passive, whereas with the Dorn Spinal Therapy, the patient has to actively co-operate to create the gentle move-

ment of the bone structure.

When clients ask if the Dorn Spinal Therapy is risky I can clearly say no, as the therapist respects the few contraindications outlined below.

There is never any risk of injuring tendons or ligaments and therefore you can repeat a treatment as often as necessary or asked for. Further on you can read what you can do yourself to promote the healing process and maintain a pain-free back.

1.2.5 Contraindications

To ensure a safe treatment and maintain a record so far of no known side effects or negative consequences due to a Dorn Treatment, every Dorn Spinal therapist has to respect the following contraindications:

- Not suitable for treatment immediately after an accident. An X-Ray has to be taken first to make sure there are no fractured vertebrae
- Spondylitis
- A treatment for a client with osteoporosis is possible but should be carried out very carefully and in constant communication with the client
- Cancer that metastasizes into the skeletal system

- Acute inflammation and fever, inflammations in the joints. The patient should wait until the inflammation is cured completely
- Acute prolapsed disc – this is a case for immediate hospitalisation!
- Paralysis, it is important to find the causes first
- Clients under constant cortisone therapy as cortisone increases the risk of bone fractures through weakening the bones
- First trimester of pregnancy or problematic pregnancies

2

DO IT YOURSELF

2.1. Building The Mental Foundation

With the following sequence of exercises you will be able to build up your own training program. Your program depends on determining which part of your body requires special care.

Of course you can do all exercises, given they are suitable for your problem. But you don't have to do all the exercises if you only want to work a certain part of your body.

Whatever you decide however, do not expect miracles - and if you do, don't forget that even miracles don't happen overnight.

However, if you stick to your exercise routine, you should feel improvements after two to three weeks. Don't stop before - ***success only comes with repetition!***

Take every little improvement as a step toward feeling better and managing your pain.

Never focus on what doesn't work but on what you have achieved. That way you can motivate yourself more and more. Even if there is no significant improvement in the first week, don't stop, because it will happen. Every person and body is different and there is no short cut to success. You just have to do it your way, but don't give up!

Self-help is possible, it just needs time and practice. The most common reasons for people not getting better are:

- Not enough practising. They try something once or twice and if it doesn't work immediately, they give up, blaming the exercises.
- They don't believe that they actually can succeed and influence their success.
- They are reluctant to take responsibility for working with and handling their own body.

Your attitude towards your pain plays a major role in overcoming back pain.

Some people tend to evaluate their condition as a catastrophe and find themselves helpless, hopeless, even useless. But they forget that there is actually a positive side to the pain which is that you can recognise it as a warning system.

Pain tells you that something in your body is wrong and that you have to take action before things start getting worse! So try taking a positive attitude towards your back pain, thank your body for telling you that something is wrong and promise your body to help it get well and healthy again. Find a positive sentence that supports your journey to well-being, one that you can remember every day at any given moment. By doing this you remain positive and that will help you overcome your pain.

Let's Talk Back

One of the most important parts in overcoming your back pain is your posture which is based on your muscular-skeletal system. By working on this system with a sequence of exercises, chances are superb that you will beat your back pain.

On the other hand, if you don't look after your posture, no exercise will work for you in the long run. Please look at yourself in a mirror and see if you are really straight, if you sit and stand upright. Sometimes, actually quite often, people feel straight but they aren't. When I get people to stand sideways to a mirror and look at themselves, they are quite surprised with what they see. So do the mirror examination now. Look at your posture from the front and the side. Recognize and determine the parts where you have to work on in the first place.

Before you start with any exercise, try and find the posture that really looks straight, even though it might feel difficult and straining initially. This is just the information you need to work on those areas, meaning stretching the related muscles, that give you the most strain.

Very often that is the chest area, where our body also holds a lot of emotions. So let the emotions run free, open up your chest, roll your shoulders back and bring your head up.

By changing your posture you might also realise that your whole organism starts working better as bad posture often

constricts organs and therefore reduces their function.

As you can see there is more than one reason to get your body straight.

2.1.1 Standing Correctly

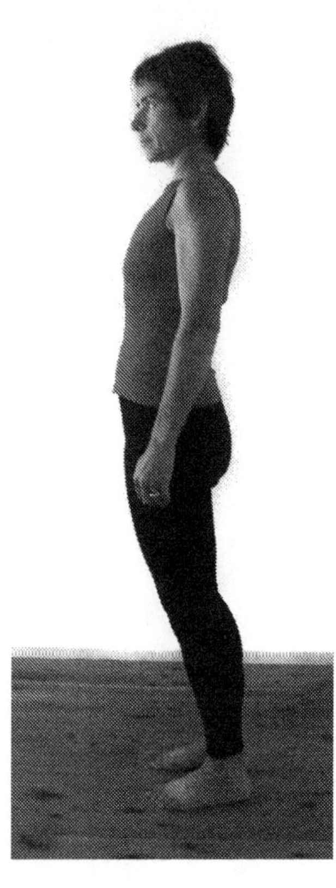

Make sure your weight is evenly spread on your feet, the balls and the heels. If you rest more on the balls of your feet, you over-stretch your knees which pushes your bottom backwards. This can produce or support a hollow back and the upper body tends to go forward to compensate the weight of the bottom half. This puts a lot of strain onto your hip joints.

If you stand more on your heels you tend to push your pelvis forward but your upper body backwards. To maintain a rather straight posture your head then comes forward which

Standing on your balls increases the lordosis and can cause pain

Standing on your heels increases upper body rounding and can cause shoulder pain and headaches as the blood flow is constricted. As you see, only minimal changes in your normal posture will have a dramatic impact on your whole body. Try to consciously take the wrong postures on your heels and balls and then the correct posture on your whole feet.

The following exercise might make it a bit easier:

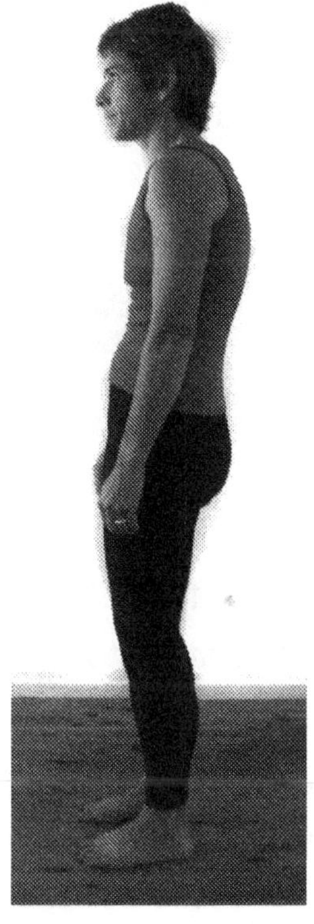

Stand with your weight evenly spread on your feet hip-width apart. Rock slowly back and forth, keeping the whole foot on the ground and experience the change of pressure under your feet. After a few repetitions rock from side to side and after a further few repetitions start circling.

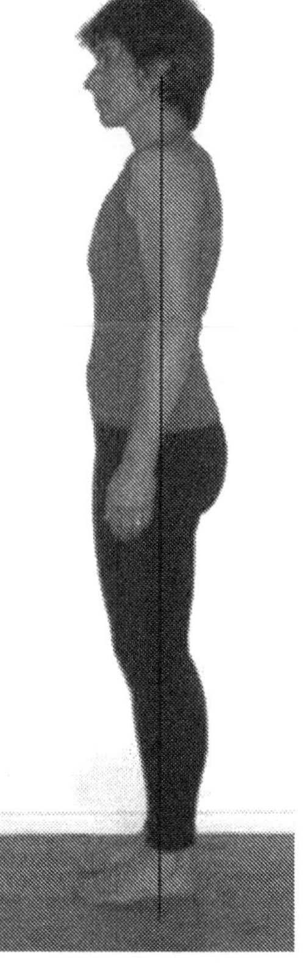

Keep your body straight the whole time and realise which muscles are used under which movement. When you get a feeling for the "centred standing position" that is how you should always stand.

Have someone look at you and make sure they can "draw" a straight line from your ear down to the pronounced bone at your foot. And then remember that position to make it your healthy position.

2.1.2 Walking Correctly

The best way to check your walking is when you walk straight towards a mirror. The heel should be the first point of contact with the ground. The toes should be directed up towards the body and you should be able to see your soles for a short moment in the mirror.

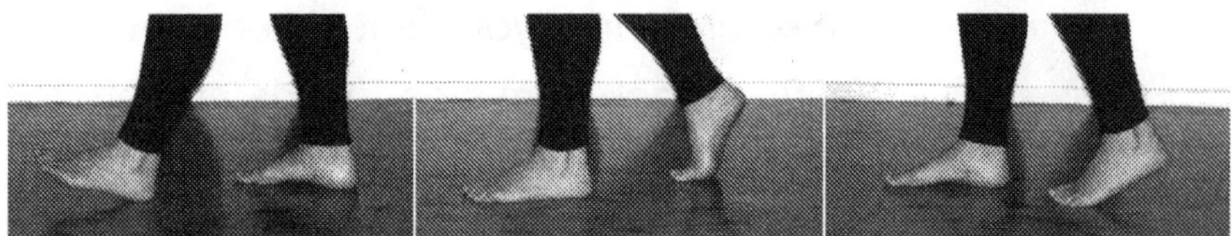

The unrolling of the foot should be happening on the lateral edge of the foot towards the ball of the foot. If you have a collapsed arch you should go and see a podiatrist to get orthotics that stabilise your arch and thereby avoid getting knee and/or lower back problems in the long run. You can check your arch in sand or with wet feet on dry ground. All you should see is the heel, the lateral edge of the foot and the balls and toes.

Once you get your feet under control, check your posture. The body should be upright, shoulders back and head up straight. Remember the position of your "standing straight" and **Face the world!**

2.1.3 Sitting Correctly

It is important to have both feet evenly on the ground to make sure the weight is evenly spread on your sitting bones and the muscles are working in balance.

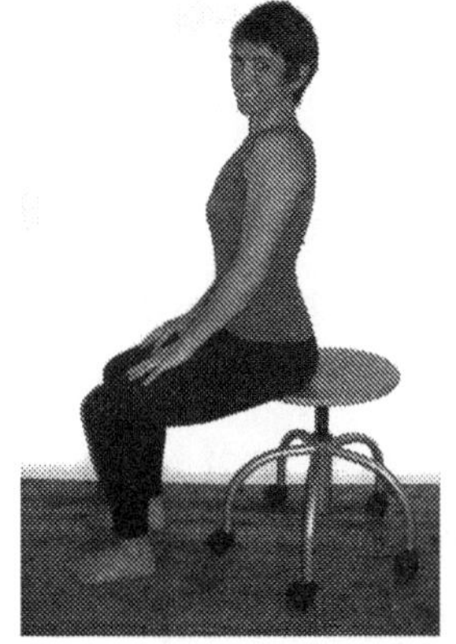
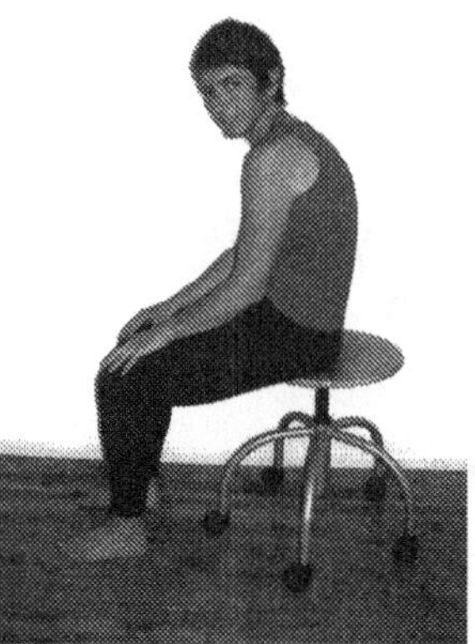
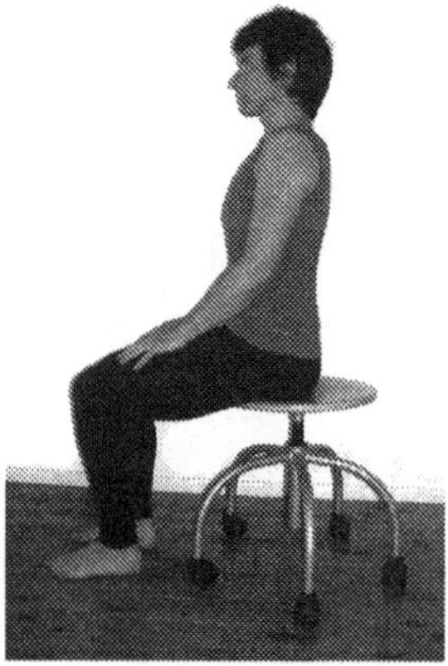

Incorrect posture *correct posture*

Make sure you are **not** arching your back too much as this position is straining for your muscular system and also leads to a hollow back.

Swap between sitting right back on the chair and using the back support and sitting further in front, using no back support but your own muscles. This change encourages different muscle sections to work instead of getting the same muscles to tense up under the constant pressure. Even slouching every now and then is allowed - providing you don't remain in that position for too long.

It is also good to use a wedge under your buttocks as that

provides a straighter position and makes it much more uncomfortable to slouch. You can purchase special wedges for a reasonable price direct from my website at www.backcaresolutions.net

2.1.4 Stress As A Cause For Back Pain

Very often back pain has nothing to do with worn or prolapsed discs, misplaced vertebrae, or different leg length but can simply be a side effect of too much stress. In that case what hurts are the muscles which are under constant tension and are forced to work in an ineffective way. It is only you who can define if stress is part of the reason for your back pain.

Warning signs in the body could be

Consequences of Stress for:	Directly Noticeable Changes	Long-Term Changes
The Body	Increased heart rate Higher blood pressure Increased release of adrenaline	Headache Stomach ulcers Increased risk of heart diseases
The Emotions	High tension Frequent frustration Easily become angry Fatigue	Strong discontentment Risk for depression Low self-esteem
The Performance	Great fluctuation Low on concentration Increased mistakes	Addictions to e.g. alcohol, nicotine, drugs
Social Environment	Increased aggressions increased reserved personality	Escalating conflicts Retreat into resignation

2.2 Self-Help Exercises

I will now explain exercises that you can do at home to support and improve your muscular-skeletal system. These exercises will reduce backaches and pain in the long run. You will learn how to balance your suspected leg length difference and reduce your headaches by bringing your aching joints back into their correct positions.

Ideally you have had a Dorn Treatment before but if not, you will still benefit from these exercises and might consider a Dorn Treatment later on.

I will also be giving you some additional acupressure points as this technique compliments the exercises. You can work on the points at any time with or without doing your exercises. By working on these points you support the energy flow that is often stagnant when pain comes up. The points are positioned on the body meridians. By looking at the pictures you will locate them very easily.

Always use the points on both sides of your body to make sure your body is in balance (e.g. left hand *and* right hand)

> ***Attention! Do not use acupressure during pregnancy as doing so might trigger labour.***

Last but not least just a few tips on how you can integrate the exercises more into your daily routine and avoid saying every day "I will do it tomorrow" and then forgetting about it:

- Before you start your working day do the exercises that are most important for you and do them again at your work place
- Repeat them before you go to your lunch break. Lunch is your reward for doing your exercises
- Have a little diary where you write down the date and time you do your exercises – and your improvements!
- Get colleagues or friends to do the exercises with you. Remember: shared fun is more fun
- Change bad habits, so use stairs instead of the lift. Walking stairs is very healthy and it always gives you a little bit of a work out. Walk to the corner shop instead of taking the car for every little distance. It also saves our environment and brings your petrol bill down.
- Take active breaks during the day, stand up and walk around, even if it's only for 2 minutes. Utilise this time for thinking if you wish.

You will notice that after a while you become really good at exercising regularly and you will miss your exercises when you don't do them. Your body will thank you.

2.2.1 Correcting The Hip-Joint

This exercise can be done whenever you feel unbalanced, are not standing evenly on both your feet or feel an ache in your hip joints. The correction should be done as often as possible during a day, 3 times each go, and it does not matter if it is done lying down or standing up.

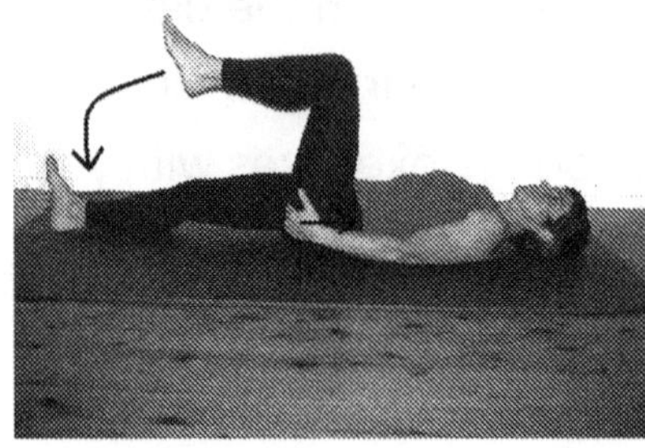

Bring the left leg into a 90° angle and place the left hand under the buttocks just where the hip joint is. The other leg remains straight.

While you pull your hand towards your head, straighten the leg and slowly lower it to the ground, similar to the movement of pushing a bicycle pedal.

Ideally you do this exercise every time you have been sitting

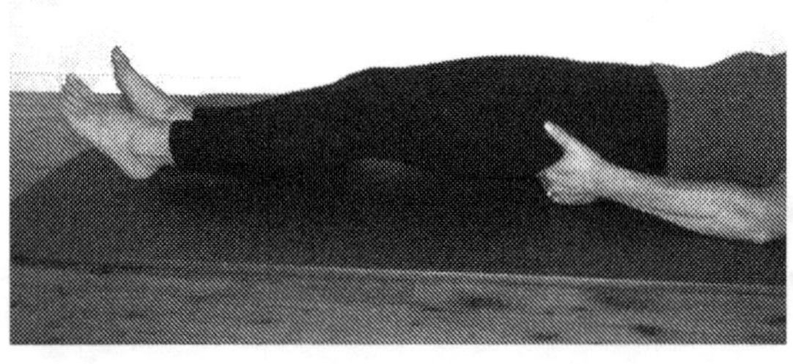

and stand up, be it from a chair, out of the car or from the lounge. And if you don't know which of your legs is the longer one just do both sides so you can be sure you have worked the correct one.

You cannot overdo this exercise!

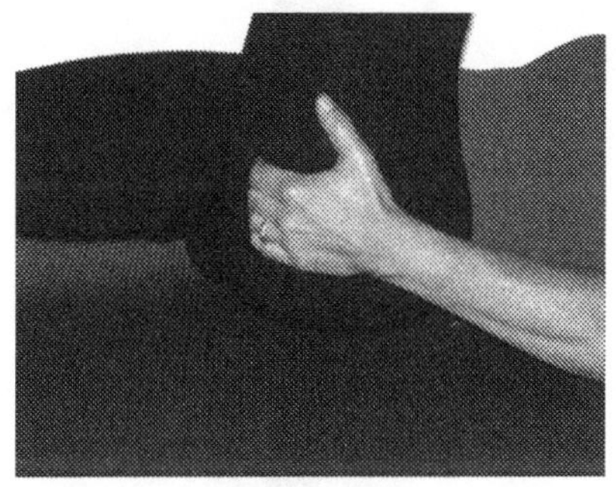

Once your joint is back in the joint socket this exercise will keep it there. Same exercise in a standing position.

You don't have to pull hard but keep the pressure up until the leg is completely straight. Take a deep breath in when you lift the leg and breathe out when you straighten it down.

If you have trouble getting your hand in place you can use a towel instead. Just roll the towel up and place it around your hip joint. Now pull with both hands on both ends of the towel whilst you slowly lower your leg.

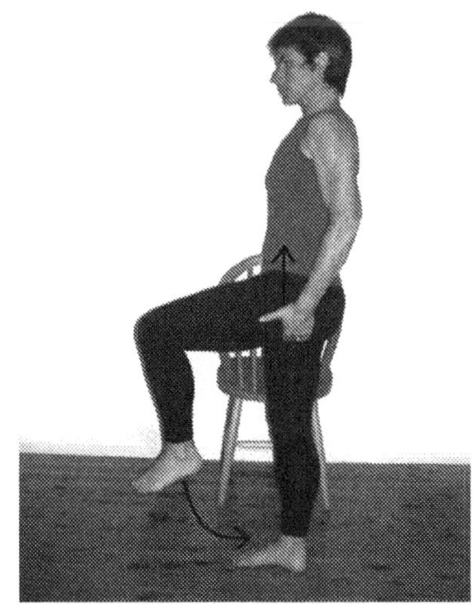

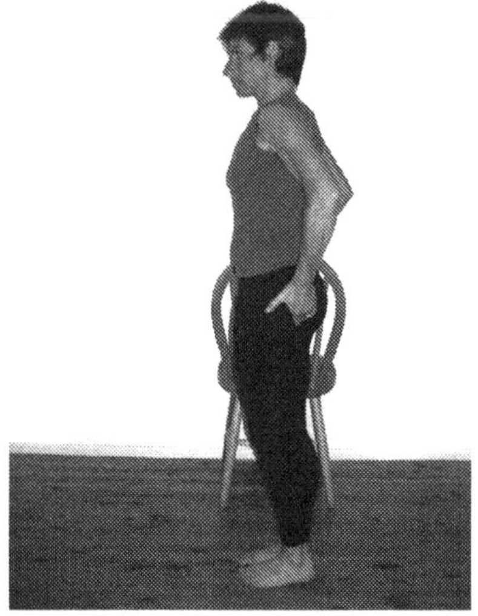

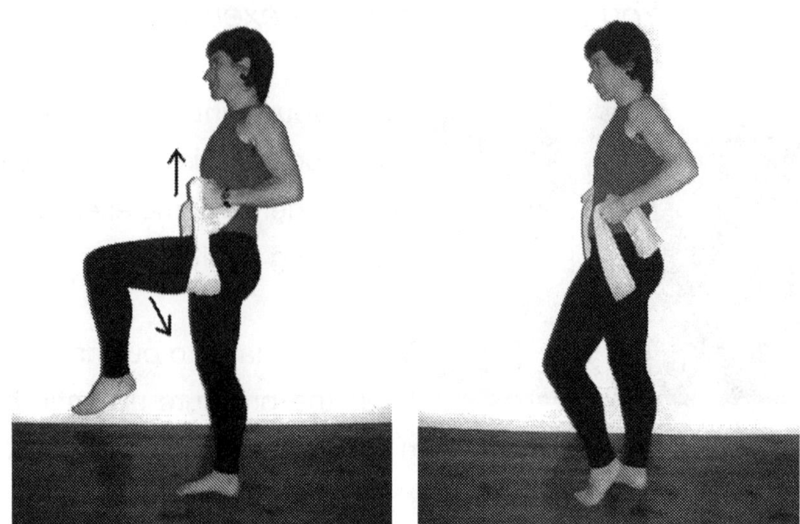

Don't forget the breathing and use this method only if you really can't reach the hip joint with your hand. Of course you can use the towel also in a horizontal position.

2.2.2 Strengthen Your Hip Area

To keep the hip joints in the right position after the correction, the muscles surrounding the joint have to be strengthened. But don't overdo it in the beginning, start easy and increase the number of repetitions of exercises slowly.

Adduction:

Stand straight and support yourself at a table or a chair with feet hip-width apart, toes pointing forward. If you want, you can stand with your static leg on a phone book or something

that elevates you a little bit to avoid “scratching” the floor when you move your other leg. Place your left hand on top of your hip.

Flex the left foot and move the leg out to the side and slowly bring it back in **without moving the torso** but imagining there is a ball between your legs that you want to squeeze together.

You should feel the hip bone move towards and away from your hand. That happens only if you keep your torso straight and don’t bend it when you move your leg.

After 5-7 repetitions change to the other side. Breathe in when you bring your leg out and breathe out when you bring it back in.

<u>Abduction:</u>

Take the same position as in the last exercise but now put strength into the outwards action.

Slowly bring your leg out, foot flexed, imagine you are pushing away a big weight, whilst breathing out, and bring it back in relaxed while breathing in.

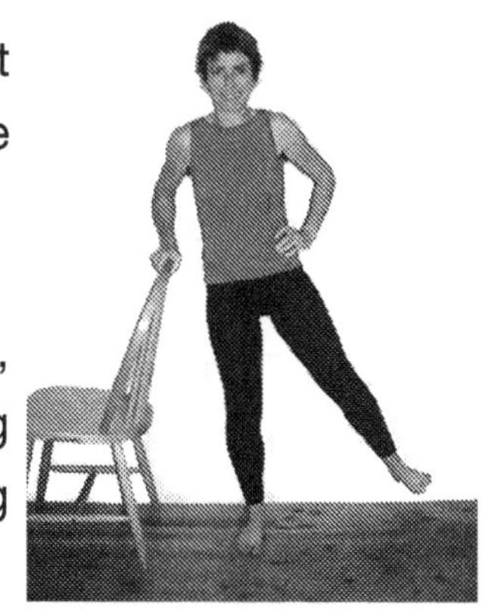

2.2.3 Retroversion Of The Femur

Stand upright and support yourself at a table or a chair, feet hip-width apart, toes forward.

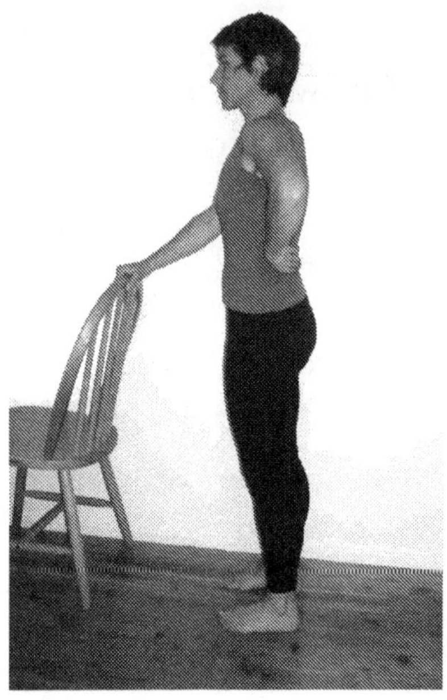

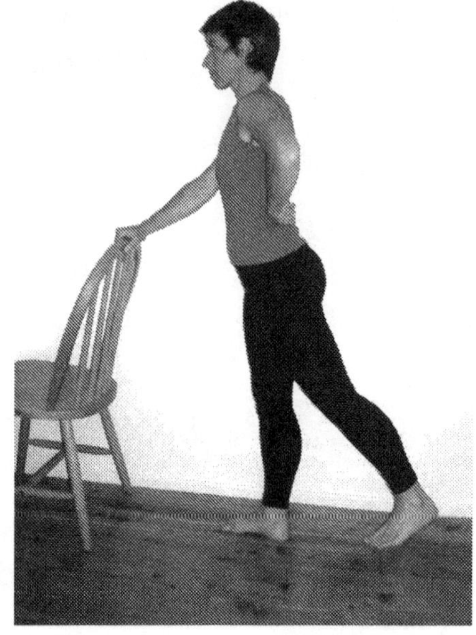

Place left hand on the lumbar spine with palms up. Bring left leg back but keep your upper body upright.

As soon as you feel the muscle of the buttocks at your hand the final position is reached and you can relax the leg. Breathe in when the leg comes forward and out on the back motion. Repeat 5-7 times and then swap sides.

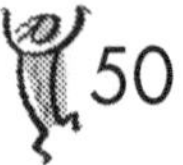

2.2.4 Stabilisation Of Your Hip With A Ball Or Folded Towel

Sit down on the frontal part of a chair with your upper body upright, feet parallel and hip-width apart, toes pointing forward.

Place a small softball or a folded towel between your knees and squeeze the ball or the towel together while breathing out. Relax and breathe in, repeat 5-7 times.

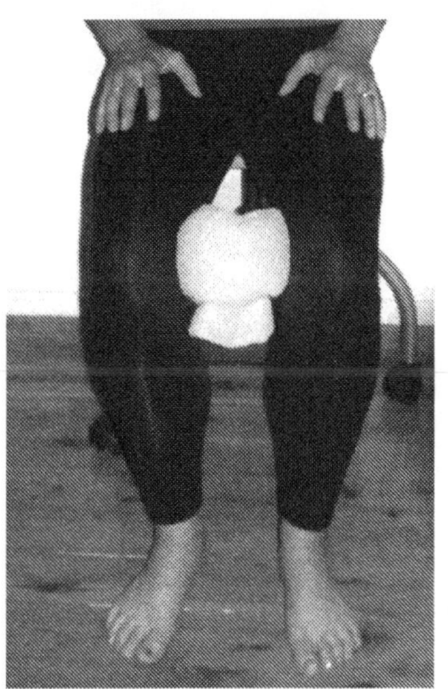

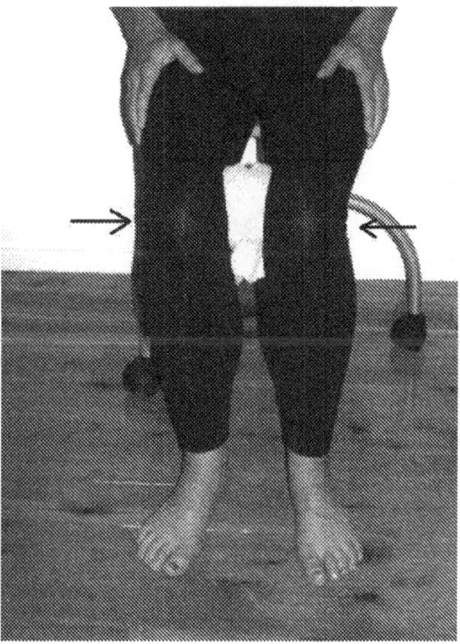

2.2.5. Knee-Bend

This exercise trains the muscles of the thigh and the ones supporting the hip joint.

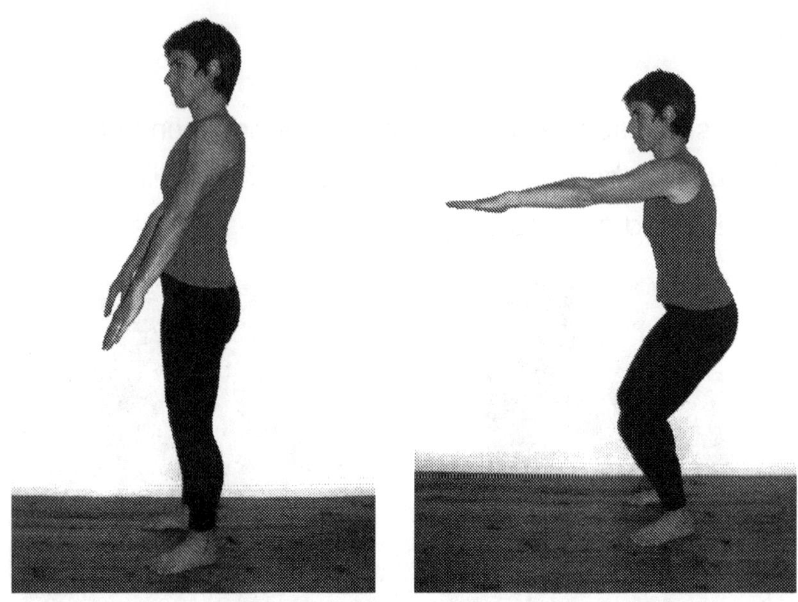

Stand upright, feet parallel but a bit more than hip-width apart. Make sure your upper body remains straight during the entire exercise and also keep your feet evenly on the floor all the time.

Slowly bend your knees and bring your arms up to chest level at the same time.

Make sure your feet remain completely on the ground, don't lift the heels. Slowly straighten your knees, bring your hands down and your pelvis forward until you reach the starting position.

Don't straighten your knees completely, always keep them slightly bent! Repeat 5-7 times, breathe in when you come up and breathe out when you go down.

This exercise is even more effective if you contract the muscles of the pelvic floor and the buttocks when you come up.

2.2.6 Mobilising The Sacro-Iliac Joint

The lower lumbar area is a very sensitive area where abnormal positions can lead to a variety of problems like joint and spinal problems, muscle tensions, pain in the groin, etc. Therefore it is good to do the exercises to prevent those and other complications and keep this area loose.

Place your right foot on a little foot stool and the left leg just a little bit backwards but straight. Make sure you keep your whole body upright during the exercise.

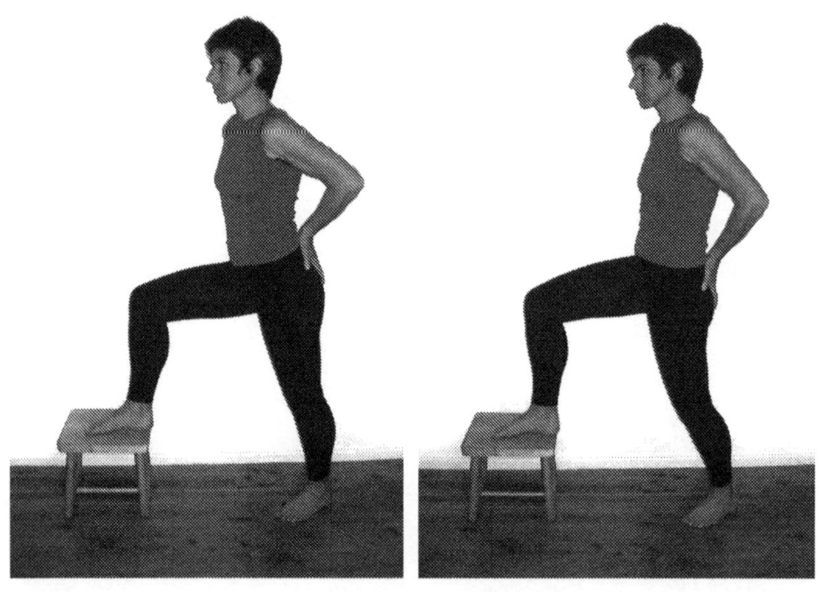

Now tip the pelvis back and forth with the right hand at the right top of the hip and the left hand just above the left buttock, following the movement of the pelvic area.

Repeat 10 times, breathe in when coming forward and out on your way back, then swap legs and do the same exercise on the other side. If you feel heat coming into the pelvic area after the exercise, you know that your circulation is working and the muscles are softening.

2.2.7 Exercise For The Sacrum

Lie flat on a mat on the floor, bring up both legs hip-width apart and at a 90° angle. Keep feet parallel and make sure the sacrum doesn't lose contact with the mat.

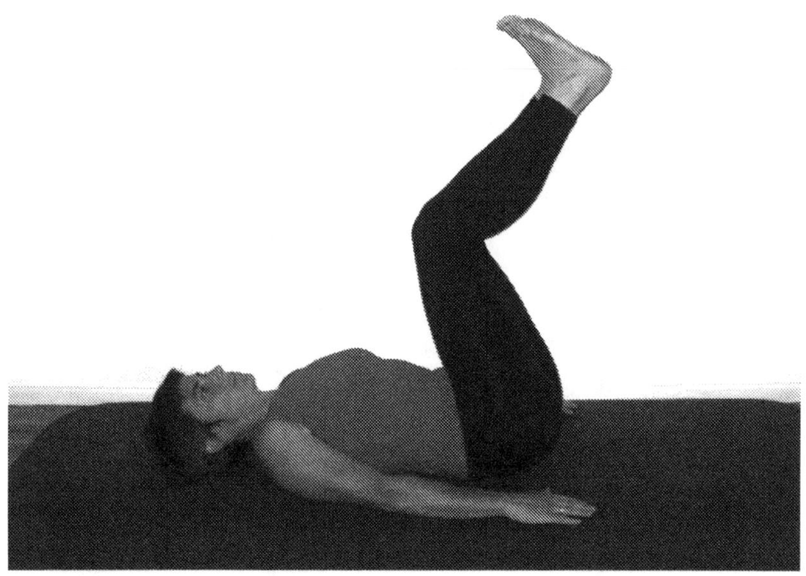

Now flex your toes towards your head and rest in this position as long as possible without straining yourself too much. Breathe evenly during the whole exercise.

If your legs start vibrating keep breathing and keep the sacrum on the floor before slowly placing your legs back down. Repeat 2-3 times, or if you have a higher fitness level then up to 7 times.

2.2.8 Balancing The Pelvic Area

Often lower back pain is related to an unbalanced pelvic area which means that the sacrum and/or the ileum are not in a straight line. That can cause restrictions in the muscles and consequently tenderness or even pain in the lower back area. A simple exercise you can do when ever and where ever will help you correct this imbalance and reduce the

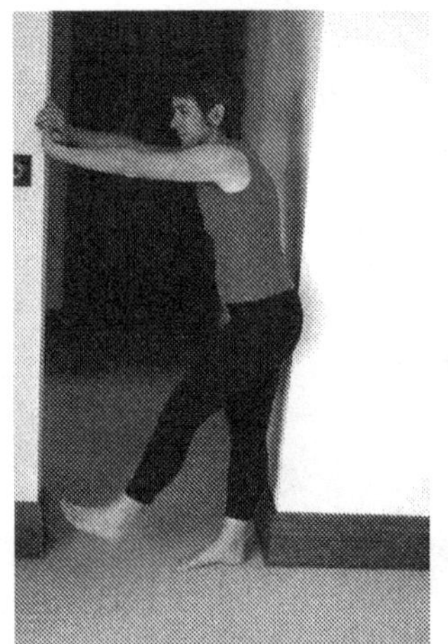

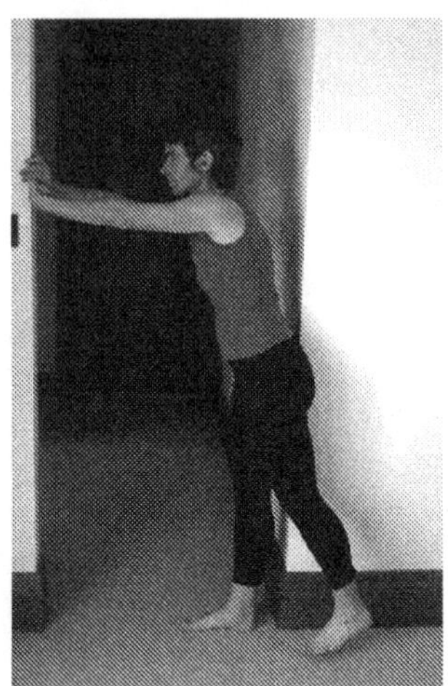

pain in that area.

Place yourself in a door frame with one side of your pelvic area touching the flat surface of the frame. Make sure it is not the spine touching the surface but just the bony area next to the spine. Let's say you place your right pelvic area at the door frame, you then hold on to the opposite door frame to make sure you are stable and able to apply some pressure. When you feel stable you start swinging your opposite leg, in this case your right leg, forward and back like a pendulum and with the back swing you increase the pressure onto your bony area. This pressure will gently move the sacrum and ileum into the right place and balance any misalignments in that area.

Do about 8 - swings on this side and then swap to the other side of the door frame to make sure you have enough swinging space for the leg.

When you lean forward slightly you can even work into the coccyx and untwist a twisted coccyx. Many of us do have a twisted coccyx from those falls onto our bottoms and it can have a great relieving effect to get the coccyx straight again. Try it, but stop if it hurts and seek professional advice.

2.2.9 Stretching The Lower Back

These stretches are very good exercises to ease the strain on the spine and to avoid a hollow back.

a) Place a pillow or a soft, folded towel over a stool. Kneel down in front of the stool and bend your upper body over it. Let your head hang down, relax and feel the stretch in the lumbar spine.

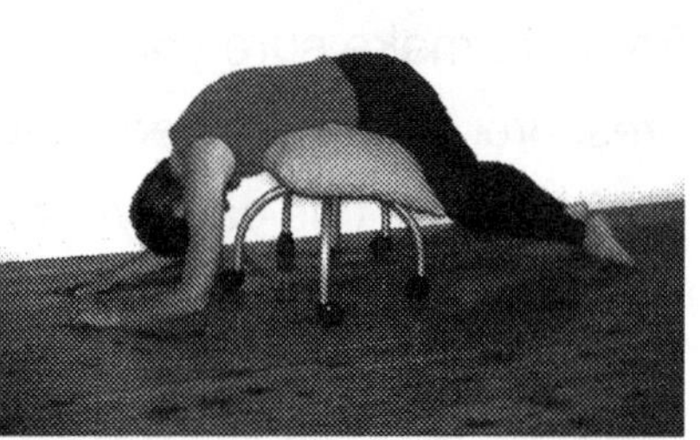

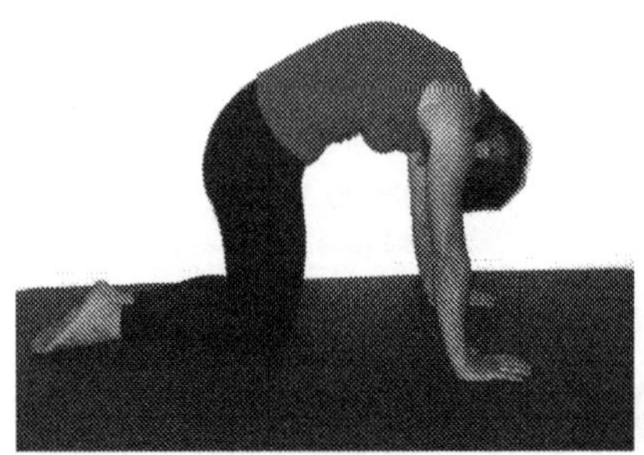

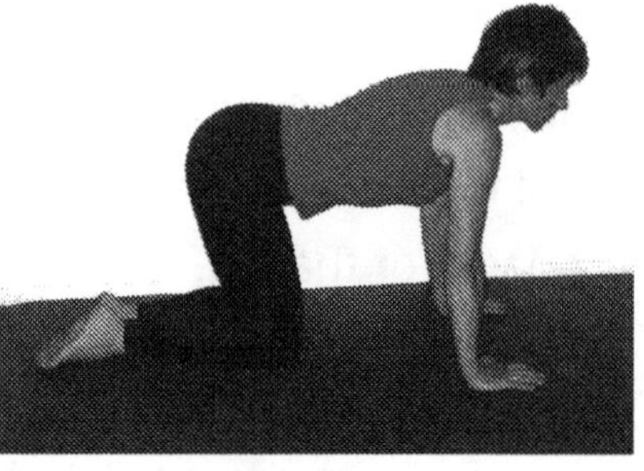

For this exercise you also can use your Swiss ball if you have one.

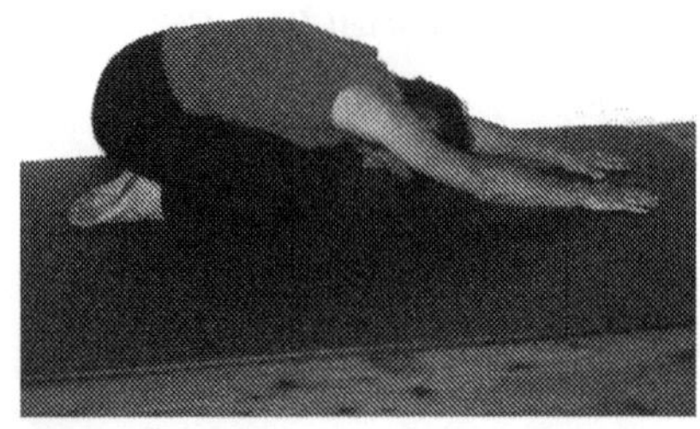

Another good stretch exercise for the lower back is the cat stand. Get down on your knees, legs hip-width apart and hands shoulder-width apart and slowly move from arched back (cat back) to hollow back. It also keeps the spine loose and is a good exercise to do at any time.

b) The next stretch is known in yoga as the "child's pose" and is very relaxing. Sit on your lower limbs, bring your arms forward until lying on your thighs with your forehead on the mat and then start walking further away with your fingers until reaching the optimal stretch.

ATTENTION!

This next exercise should only be done if you don't have any problems with your lumbar spine. If you have a protruding lumbar vertebra or lower back pain, only do the exercises a and b above.

Because you are bending forward with your head down, in this next exercise, you need to be aware that this will send more blood to your head. If you feel dizzy, stop the exercise immediately as you might lose balance and hurt yourself.

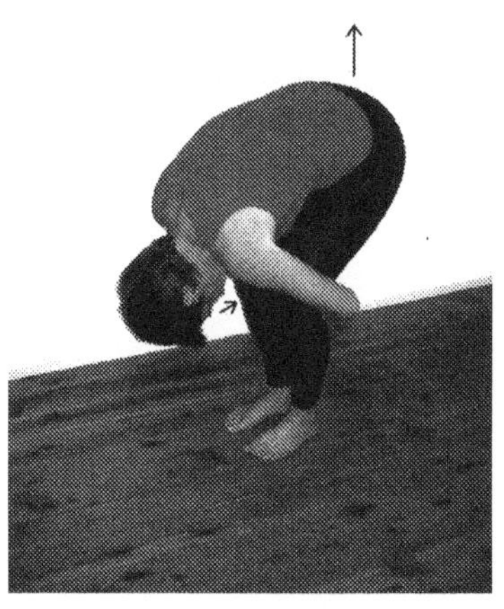

Stand straight with feet parallel and slightly apart, bend the upper body over, relax your head and place the lower arms around

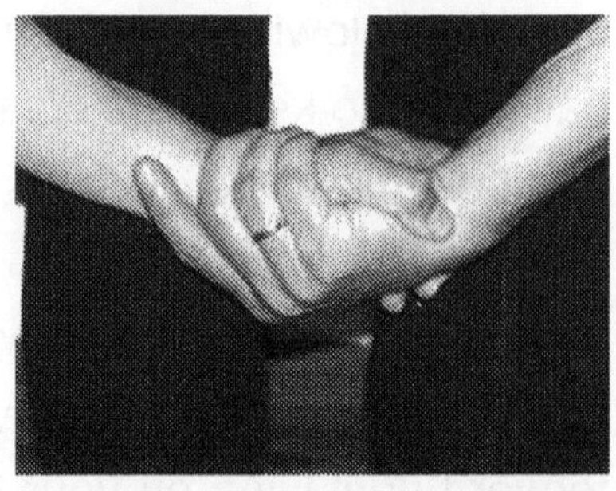

the back of your bent knees until you can hold your hands as shown in the picture on the right.

Now push upwards by trying to straighten your knees as far as possible while still keeping your hands clasped. Hold this position for a few seconds, relax without getting up, and repeat the pushing 5-7 times.

You should not hold this exercise for much longer than 20 seconds and make sure the knees are bent without pointing inwards.

When you have finished the exercise, let go of your hands and slowly roll yourself up, one vertebra after another, head last.

To get the most benefit out of this exercise you should follow with the hip correction exercise just in case the hip joint might have moved. Try to breathe deep into the lumbar spine and the sacrum.

2.2.10 Knee Joint

If you suffer from knee pain, or after having corrected your hip joints, you still feel uneven, you can do the following exercise to correct your knee joint.

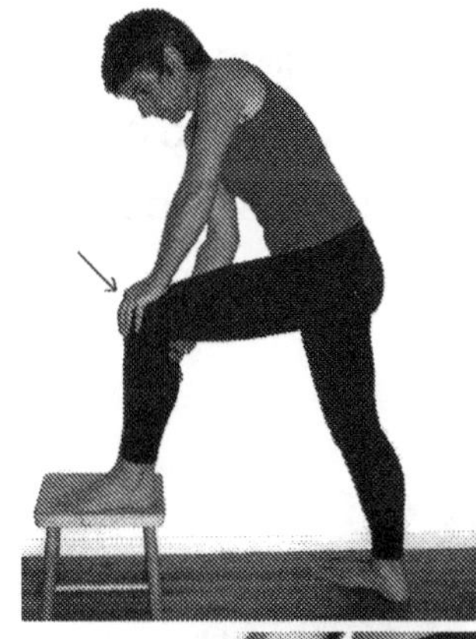

This exercise is performed standing up. Bend your knee to a 90° angle. Ideally you place the leg that needs correction on a foot stool or something else that brings it up a little bit higher.

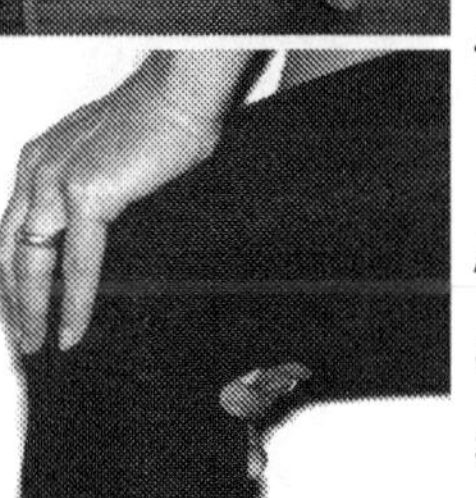

Then you place one hand on the patella (knee-cap), the other underneath the knee to support it.

Apply some pressure on the knee and while keeping the pressure up, straighten the leg.

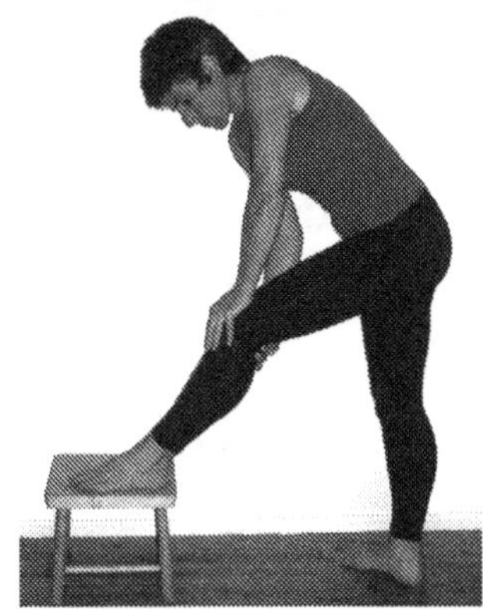

Repeat it three times and swap legs to make sure you have corrected the right one. If you do this exercise to reduce pain in your knee you only do the knee that hurts. But also have a look in the section 3.1 "Acupressure Points" in this book for complementary acupressure.

To avoid any overstretching of the leg, make sure that the calf-hand supports the knee and do the exercise carefully.

2.2.11 Ankle Joint

Pain in the ankle joint or feeling shaky when walking can be signs of a wrongly positioned ankle joint which can also cause a difference in leg length. Here is an easy exercise you can use any time you suspect a problem in your ankle joint.

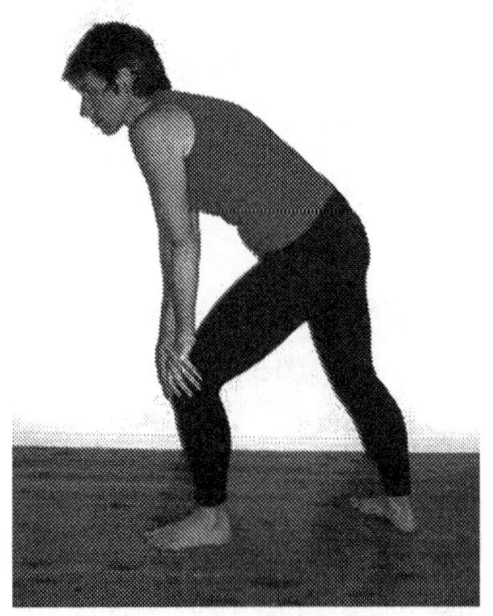

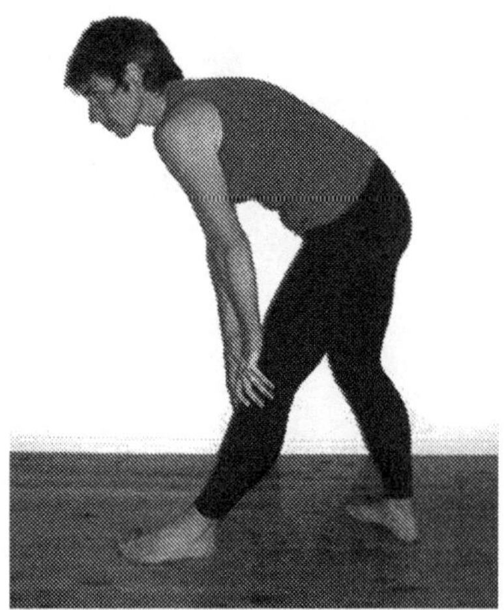

Bring the foot you want to work on in front, place both hands on top of the knee and with a rocking movement go back and forth, keeping the pressure up. You can also do it without your hands on the knee, just a nice rocking movement with your weight on the rocking foot.

The sole of the foot remains completely on the floor during the entire exercise. Repeat 5-7 times and swap to the other leg.

Be careful that you don't overstretch the leg and make sure you are not doing any jerky moves.

Another good exercise is to simply walk backwards as this trains muscles and ligaments in the joints even more so.

2.2.12 Swinging Your Arms

This exercise is particularly good for anyone sitting the whole day and tightening up in the upper body. It relaxes and regulates the thoracic spine and is easy to do at any time and place.

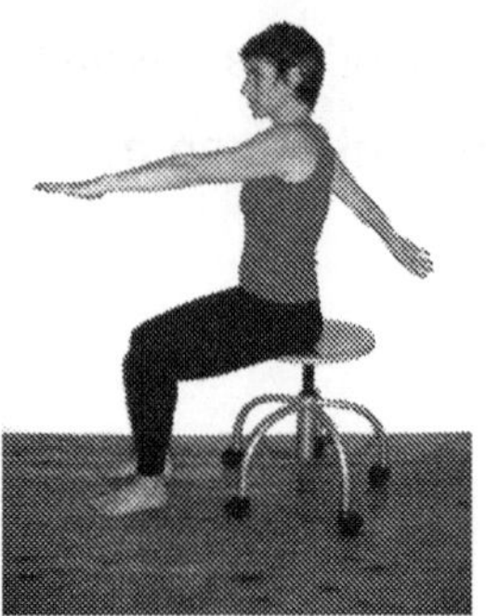

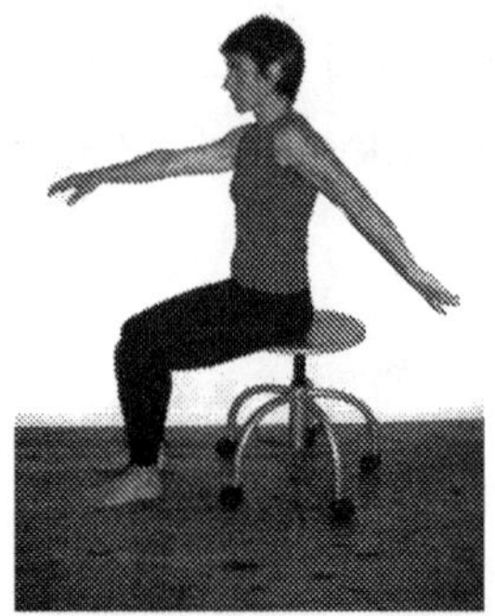

Sit upright on your stool, legs hip-width apart in a 90° angle, both feet completely on the floor. Now alternatively, loosely swing your arms forwards to shoulder height and backwards, fully extended. Keep your arms straight but not tight and work out of the shoulders not the elbows. Breathe in and out very deeply.

2.2.13 Stretch The Upper Body

a) Bring both your arms straight back, interlock your hands and rest them in the middle of your buttocks. Once you are comfortable in that position, bring your shoulders back and start pulling your arms evenly down. Feel how the chest opens up and your body becomes straighter. Relax and repeat 5-7 times.

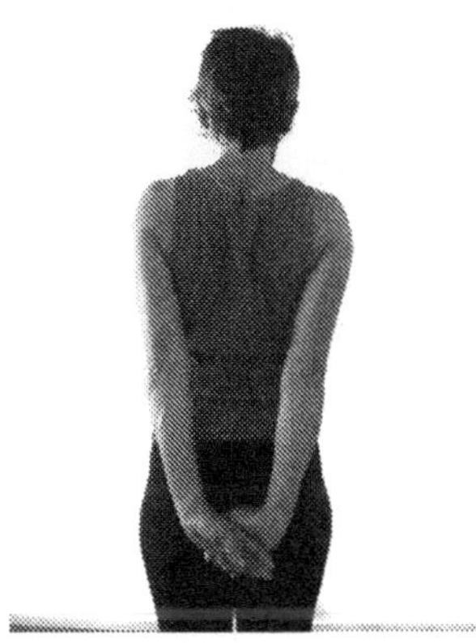

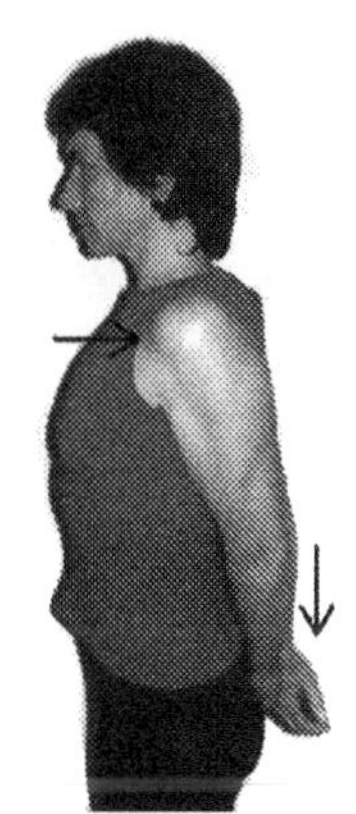

b) Find somewhere to hold on to, like the edge of a cupboard, a pole, a tree, the wall, etc. Hold with one hand and start walking away from your arm in a circular movement while still holding on until the stretch is the strongest. Hold for 20 seconds and walk back. Relax and repeat 3-5 times, then swap arms.

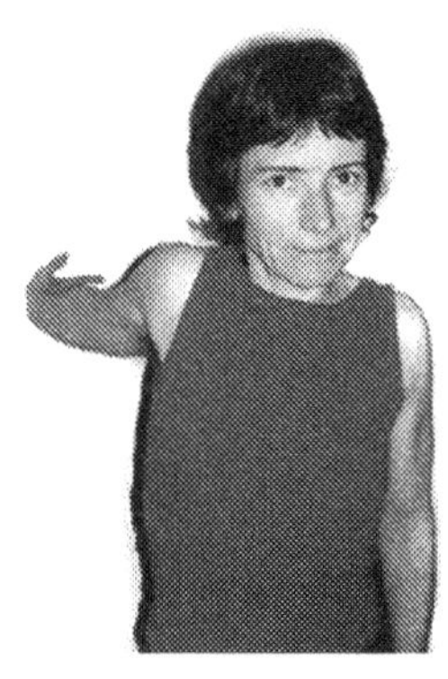

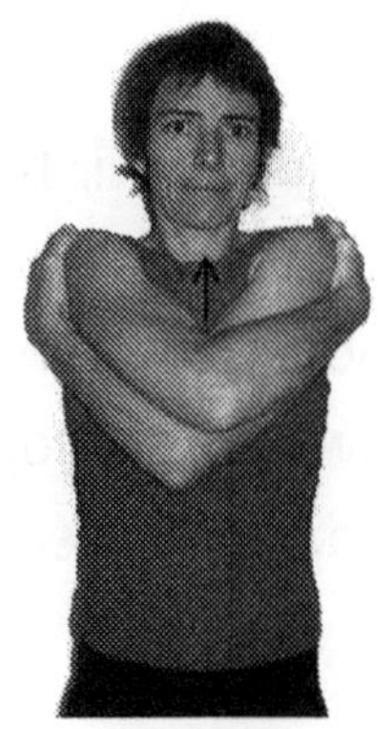

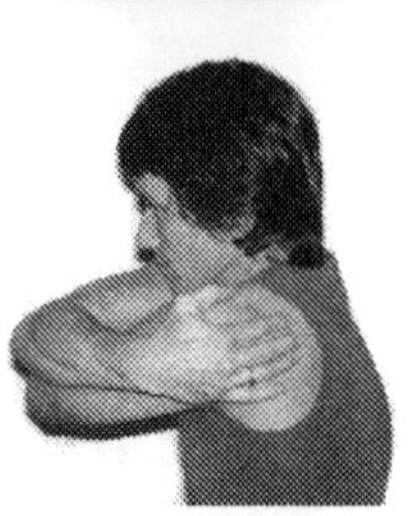

c) Give yourself a hug around the shoulder blades, as far as possible. Then slowly lift up your arms and at the same time start bending your back. Breathe out when lifting and in when relaxing.

Feel the stretch in the upper back, hold for 20 seconds, relax and repeat 5-7 times.

Pull up and forward as if describing a half circle, feel the stretch between the shoulder blades.

2.2.14 Straightening Of The Upper Body

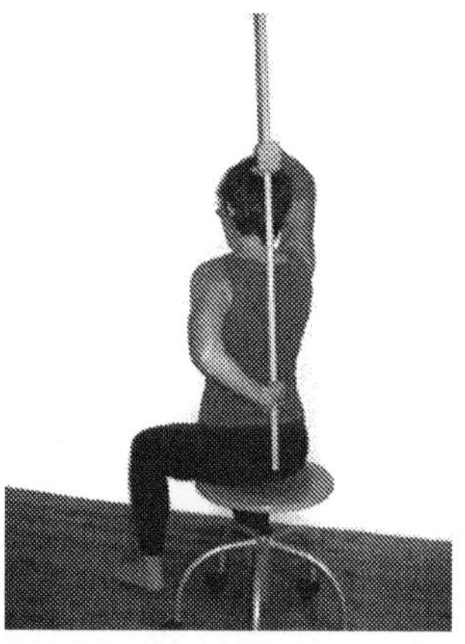

Take a broom stick or any other straight stick. Sit on the front part of a chair, hold the stick on your back where the spine is. With a straight back lean forward and stand up off the chair making sure the stick keeps touching the spine all the time. This exercise sounds much simpler than it really is, but keep trying. If it's really hard to keep touching the spine it just means that your chest muscles are too tight and you have to stretch them more regularly.

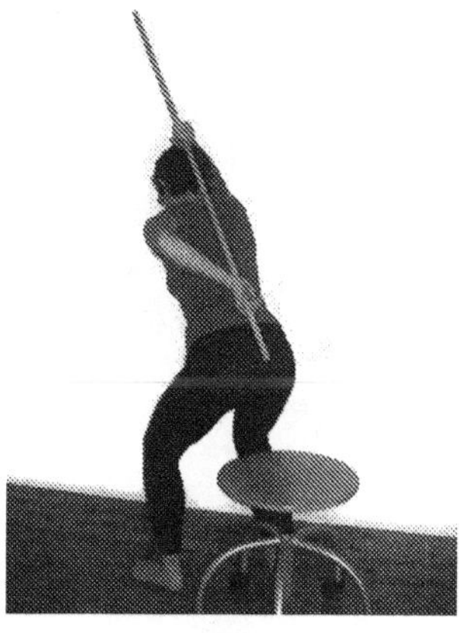

Now take the stick, bring it behind your back in a horizontal way and wrap your arms around it. This can proof difficult when your chest and upper arm muscles are very tight. But keep trying. The best time to do this exercise is when watching TV or sitting at the table talking. Keep the stick as long as you feel comfortable. The more often you do these exercises the more straighter you will feel.

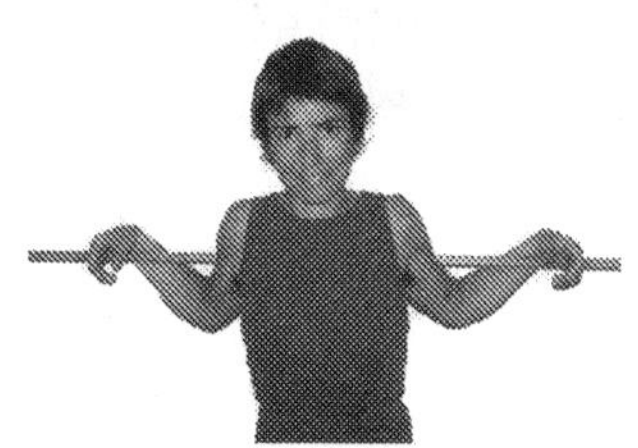

After you have finished with those exercises it is a good idea to simply stretch your arms towards the ceiling making sure your body is straight or even slightly bent backwards. That will release the tension that can build up when you "hang over the stick". And it is a real feel good stretch. Imagine you are trying to pick the highest hanging cherries in the tree.

2.2.15 Self Massaging Of The Trapezius

The Trapezius, the muscle that runs across your shoulder, is probably the most tense muscle in most people. Therefore it is good to know an effective self-massage that you can use on a regular basis. You have probably already done a similar movement when ever you feel tight in your shoulder area but there is a simple trick to make this massage work more effectively.

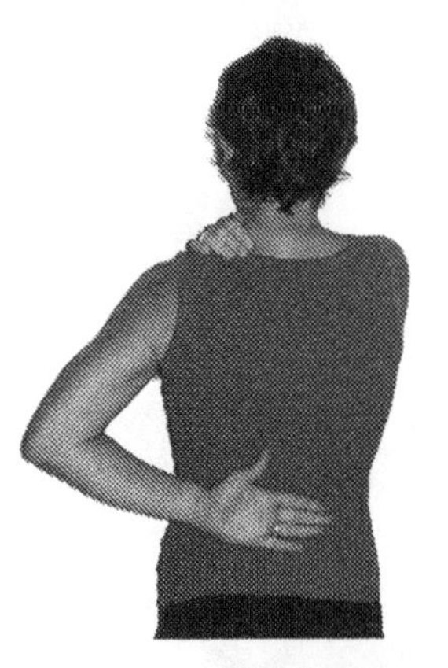

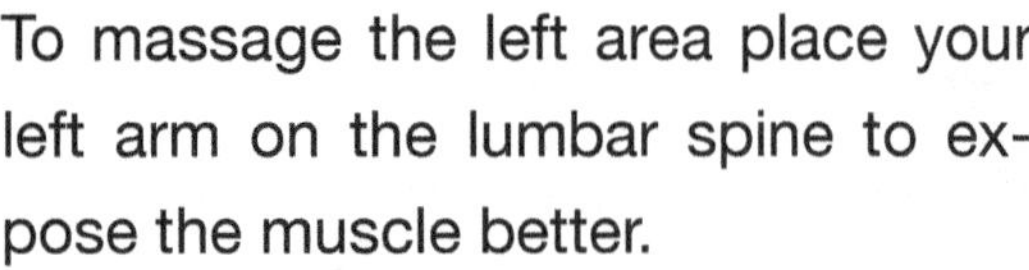

To massage the left area place your left arm on the lumbar spine to expose the muscle better.

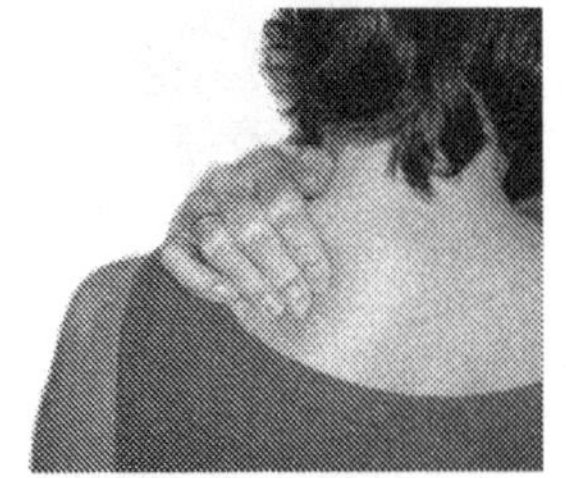

With the right hand massage the muscle in a rotating motion and/or pull it forward with your fingertips. Swap sides.

2.2.16 The Jaw Joint

Do you have problems with chewing, tension in the jaw muscles, pain opening or closing your jaw or even untreatable headaches?

One reason can be a wrongly positioned denture where teeth do not sit properly on top of each other. So have them checked by your dentist. If that is okay maybe the following exercises can help you, given you do them every day 3-5 times. It just takes a couple of minutes all together.

Open your mouth as far as possible. Take your face in your hands and have the tip of your index finger resting in the jaw joint. The thumb is under the lower jaw along the bone line.

Now push the jaw slightly back and up towards the nose. Resist the push and close your mouth slowly. Just before you close your mouth completely push your palms in and up.

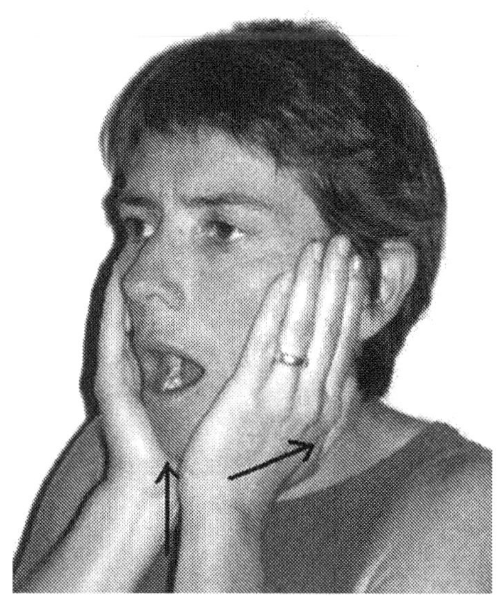

2.2.17 Massage Of The Masseter Muscles

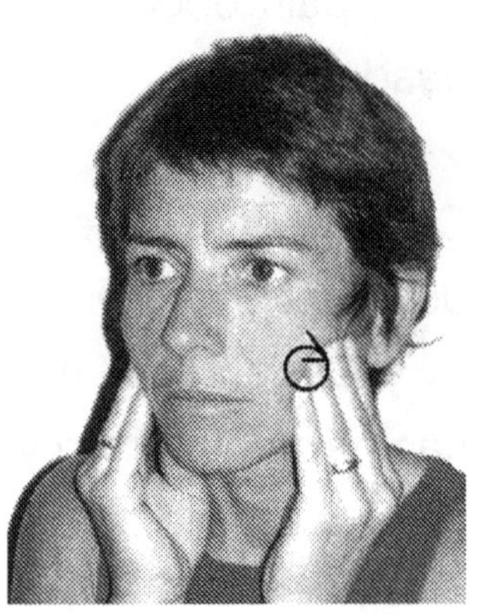

With the tips of your fingers on the cheeks and just under the cheekbones, massage the muscles in rotating motions.

Use your voice during the massage, humming brings more relaxation. And with a slightly open mouth it might be even more relaxing.

2.2.18 Exercise For The Thighs

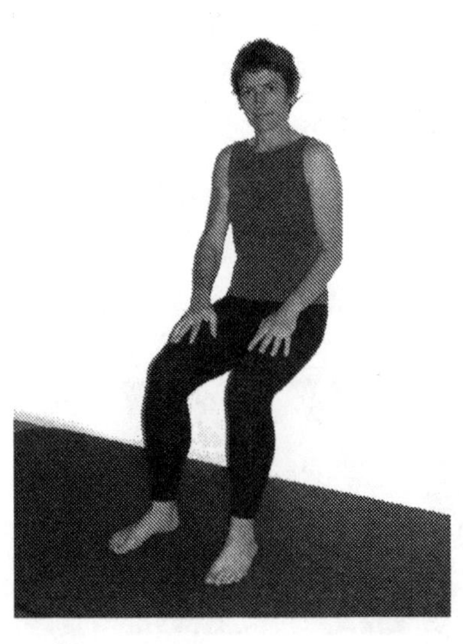

Strengthening the muscles of your back, buttocks and legs
The stronger these muscles, the straighter your posture, the less back problems you will experience. So it is good to get into a routine to work these muscles constantly.

Lean with your back against a wall, feet hip-width apart and about a step away from the wall, knee and feet in one line, shoulders and head touching the wall.

Slowly slide down the wall bending your legs to a 90° angle without losing contact with the wall. Remain in this position until you feel the strain in your thighs.

Make sure you are not moving your knees in or out. The more bent the legs are, the more intensive the training is. When you can't hold it anymore slide up again, shake the legs and repeat the exercise. When you have finished the exercise stretch your thighs.

2.2.19 Stretching The Thighs and Groin

Hold on to the wall, a chair, or anything stable and with the other hand hold your foot and bring it up towards the buttocks.

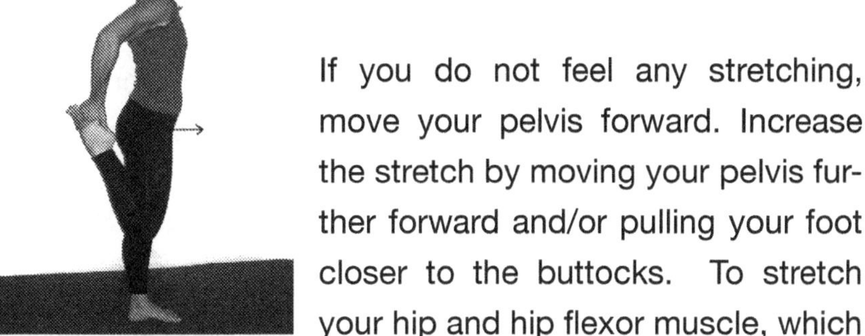

If you do not feel any stretching, move your pelvis forward. Increase the stretch by moving your pelvis further forward and/or pulling your foot closer to the buttocks. To stretch your hip and hip flexor muscle, which often are very tight in people who sit a lot, and can contribute to lower back pain, take the same starting position but when bringing the leg up extend it back and feel the stretch in your groin area.

You can also use a towel instead of your hand. This allows you to move your leg further back and increase the stretch.

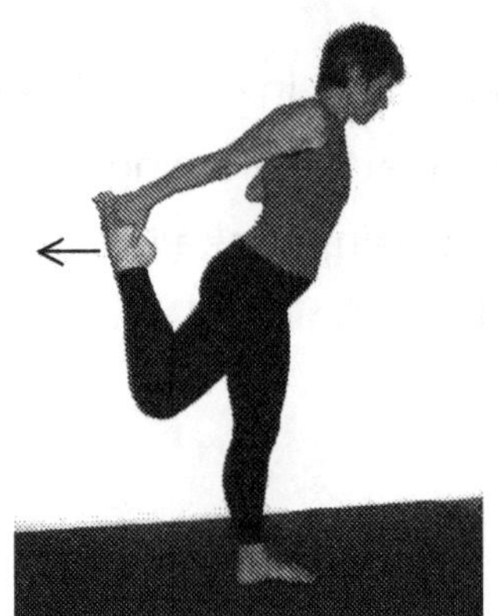

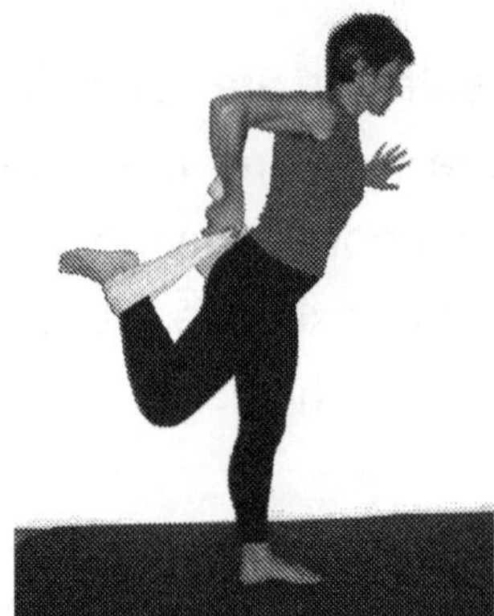

2.2.20 Exercises For The Muscles Of Your Back And Buttocks

a) Use a soft surface like grass or a rubber mat, bring yourself into a cat-stand, keep your back straight with your nose pointing towards the floor.

Now stretch your right arm forward and at the same time your left leg straight back with the foot turned out. This will strengthen the muscles of your buttocks. Keep your arm, head, back and leg all in one straight line.

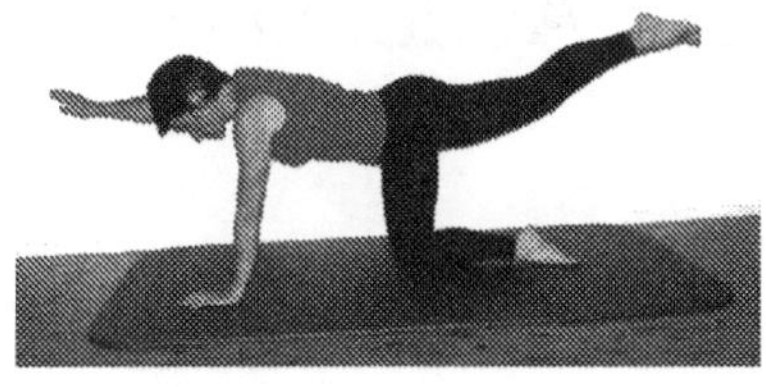

Hold for 20-30 seconds and then swap sides, left arm and right leg. Repeat 5-7 times.

If you feel problems in your wrists make sure you do the exercise for the correction of the wrists afterwards - see section 2.2.24.

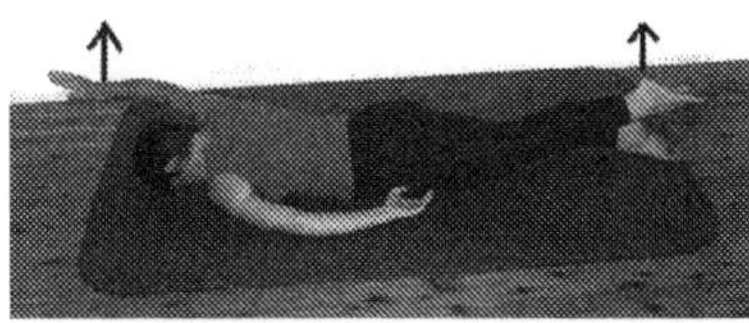

b) Lie flat on your stomach, nose pointing down and left arm alongside your body.

Lift your head slightly, stretch your right arm straight forward and at the same time lift your left leg and stretch it straight back. Hold for 20-30 seconds and then swap sides.

Repeat 5-7 times. Stop the exercise immediately if you feel pain in your lower back.

To make it even harder you can lift both arms and legs at the same time. The further you lift them from the floor, the better the training.

Make sure to loosen your body after the exercises by shaking it and swinging your arms and legs.

2.2.21 Strengthening Your Abdominal Muscles

This is vital to avoiding back problems, as a strong muscular system in the abdominal and stomach area supports your back and your spine as do the back muscles. If you look at both systems working together it is like a strong corset holding your spine in the right position.

Apart from that it helps you look good - and if you look good, you are more likely to present yourself to the world in an upright posture. Your back will be grateful.....

a) Straight muscles
Lie down on your back on a soft mat, bend your knees but with feet on the floor parallel and hip-width apart, arms alongside.

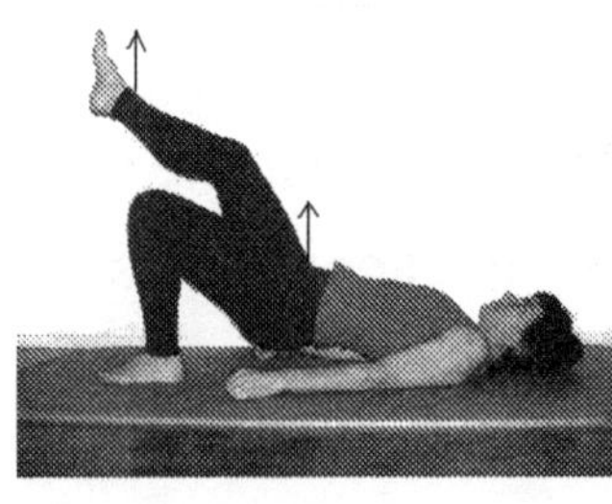

Pull your chin towards your chest and make sure your head rests on the floor during the exercise. Lift up your pelvis as far as possible, contract your abdominal muscles and bring up one leg, hold for a few seconds, lower it down and bring the other one up.

Keep going until you realise you have let go of the contraction. Breathe in when lifting and breathe out when lowering

the leg. Relax and repeat 5-10 times.

Lie flat on the floor, bring your legs in to a 90° angle, pull your chin to the chest and place your arms alongside. To stabilise your legs you can cross your feet over, depending on what works better for you.

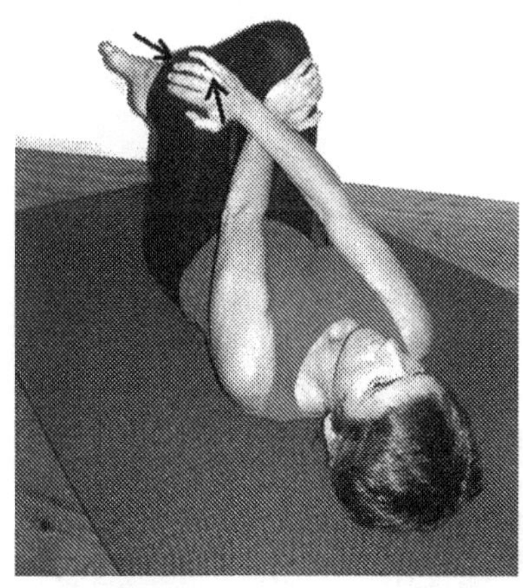

Now place your left hand on the right thigh just above the knee, and the right hand on the left leg. Press your palms onto the thighs and at the same time resist the pressure with your legs.

Hold for a few seconds, relax and repeat 10-15 times. It is important to keep breathing during the exercise, so breathe out when you press against your knees and breathe in when you relax.

b) **Oblique muscles**

Again lie flat on your back on a mat, stretch your cervical spine and keep your head on the ground.

Bring both legs into a 90° angle and cross your feet. Place your left palm on the right thigh and push against the leg while withstanding the pressure with the leg. Hold for a few seconds, breathe and relax, before swapping sides.

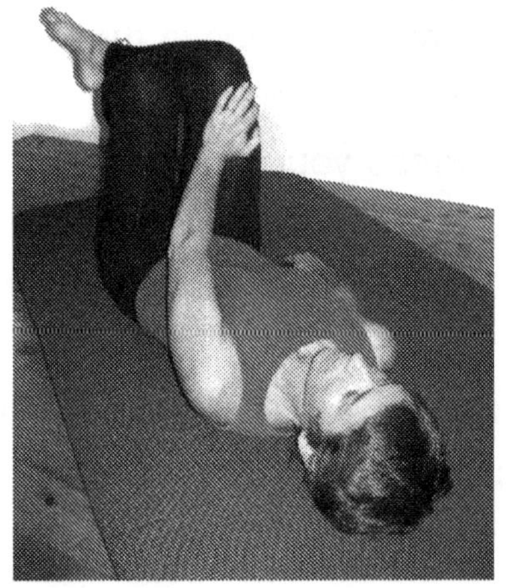

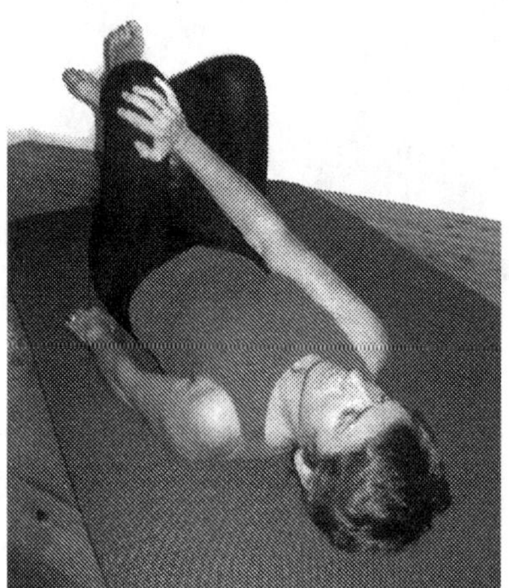

Repeat both sides 10-15 times.

2.2.22 Strengthening Your Neck Muscles

Place your palm on your forehead, apply pressure to the forehead but withstand the pressure.

Relax and repeat 10-15 times

With your right palm apply pressure to your right temple, and at the same time resist with your head. Relax and repeat 10-15 times. Repeat on the other side.

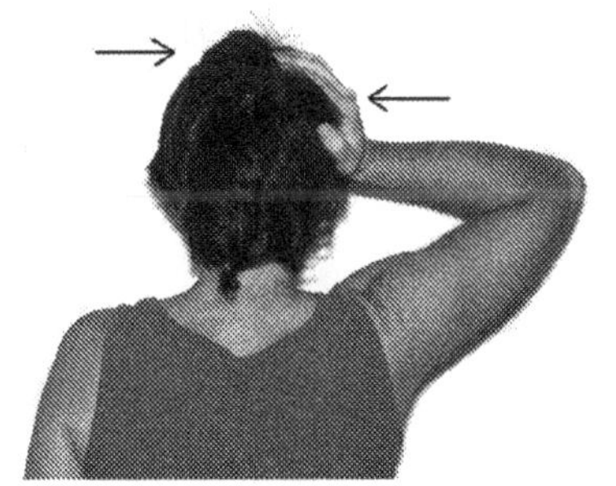

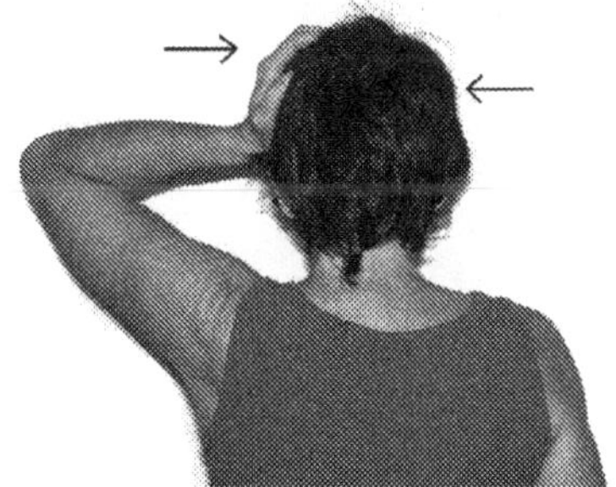

2.2.23 Stretching Your Neck Muscles

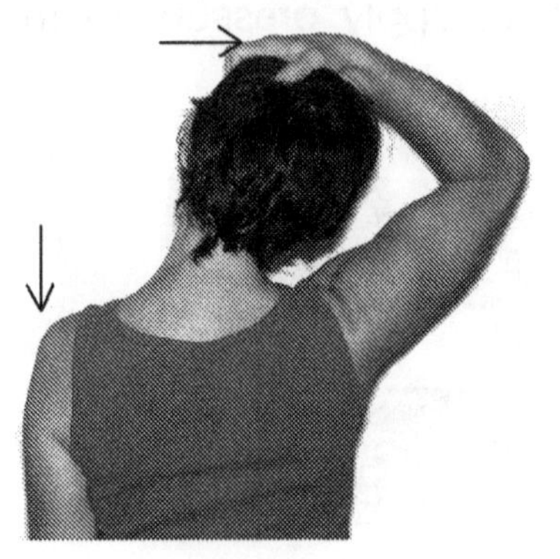

These exercises are very important to repeat at various times during the day, particularly when sitting at computers or desks for a long time, and for people with tight shoulder and neck areas.

Place your right hand over your head onto your left temple, pull gently towards the right shoulder and at the same time pull the left hand towards the floor.

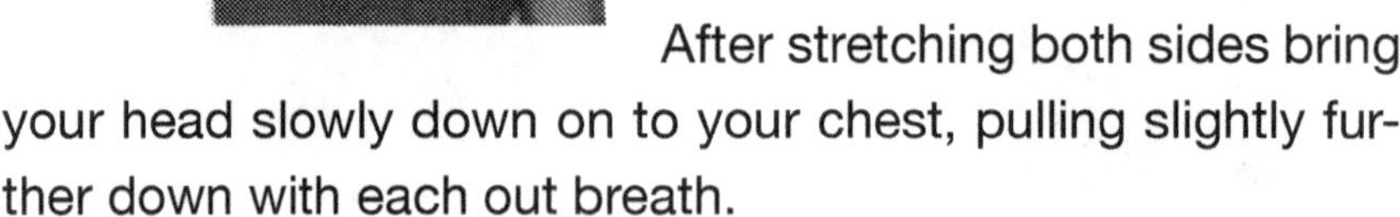

When you feel the stretch, hold it for 15 seconds before relaxing and swapping sides.

After stretching both sides bring your head slowly down on to your chest, pulling slightly further down with each out breath.

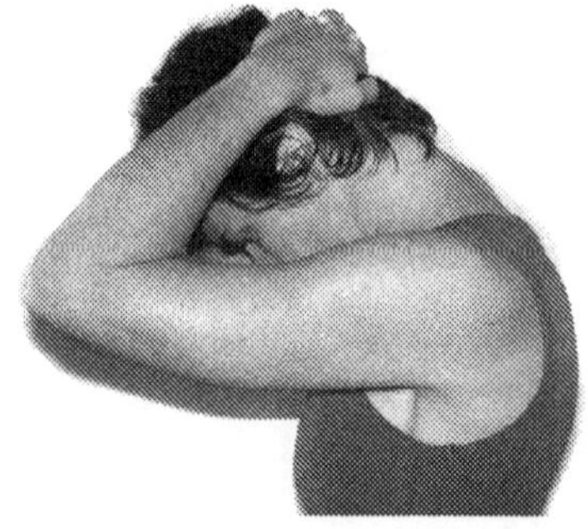

Relax a little bit when you breathe in and take it even further down with the next out breath. That gives a good stretch to your posterior neck muscles. Repeat 5-7-times.

2.2.24 Working On Your Cervical Spine

When your neck feels tight and aching, maybe even accompanied by a slight headache, you can try and correct your cervical spine yourself. It is important to work on both sides of the spine as you can't know which side is affected.

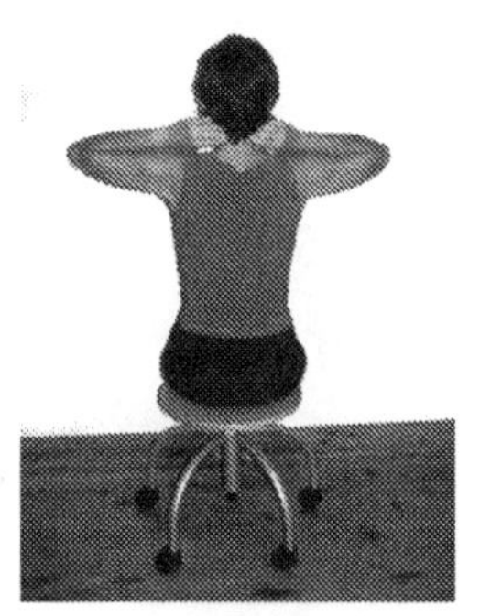

Place the tips of your fingers next to your cervical spine along the crease. Push your fingertips towards the spine while turning your head from side to side in a "no" saying motion.

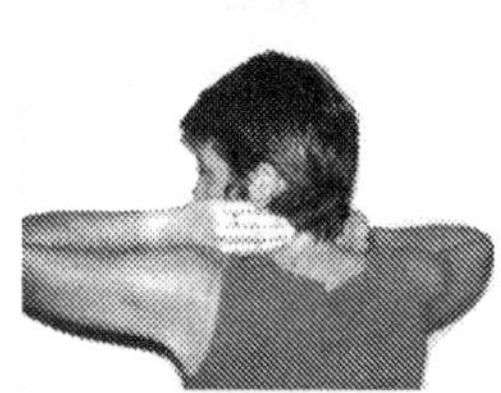

When you feel an imbalance, one side tighter than the other, remain on that particular spot, press a little bit harder towards the spine while still moving your head.

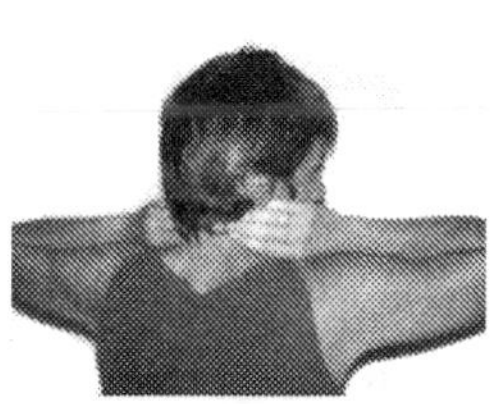

Always respect any pain and don't press too hard!

Relax And Loosen Your Neck

Let your head come forward on your chest and roll it a few times from right to left before going into a full circling movement, clockwise and counter-clockwise.

This is a good relaxing exercise when you work a lot in front of a computer.

2.2.25 Work All Your Other Joints Where You Feel Stiffness, Pain Or Pressure

Whenever there is any sort of ache or pain in your joints anywhere in your body, it is good to know that you can try an easy exercise as a first step.

Often, pain in the joints is a consequence of wrongly positioned joints, just as it is in the spine. This can of course happen in any joint in the body such as fingers, elbows, wrists, toes, etc.

To get relief from this pain we always follow the same principle: bring the joint back into the correct position. If that doesn't reduce the pain, there is obviously another problem that is creating the pain!

How do we do the joint movement?

Little joints like fingers or toes:

Hold on to the bone closest to the sore joint, push towards the joint and under pressure bend it to 90°.

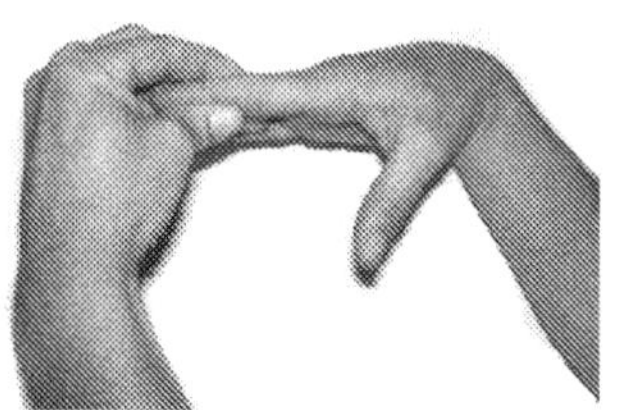

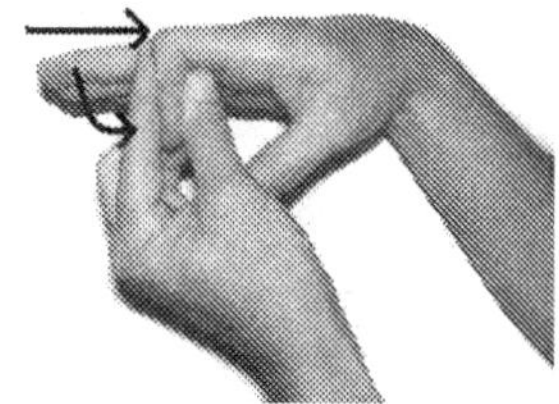

Wrist joint:

Hold your hand just above the wrist joint, push back towards the joint and move down until reaching a 90° angle. Repeat 3-5 times.

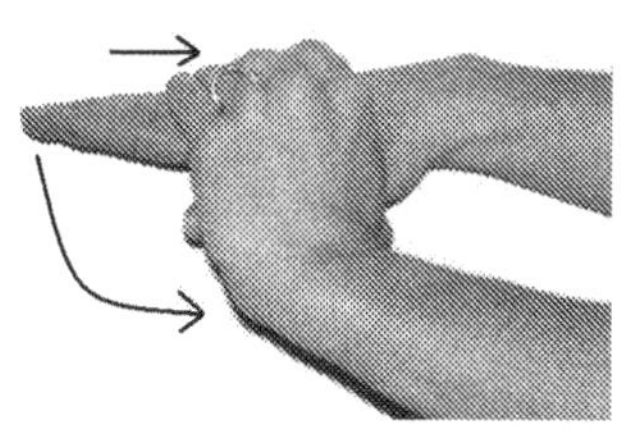

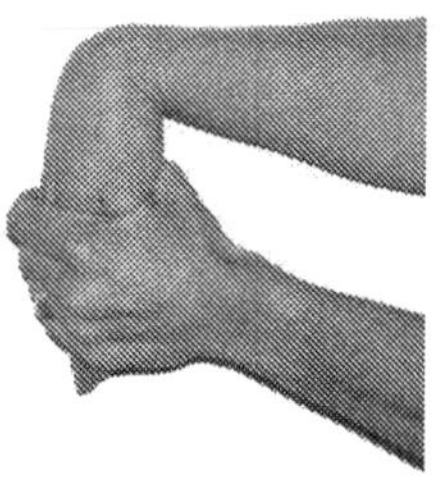

Elbow joint:

Bring your arm into a 90° angle, hold the wrist and apply pressure onto the elbow joint while straightening the arm. Repeat 3-5 times.

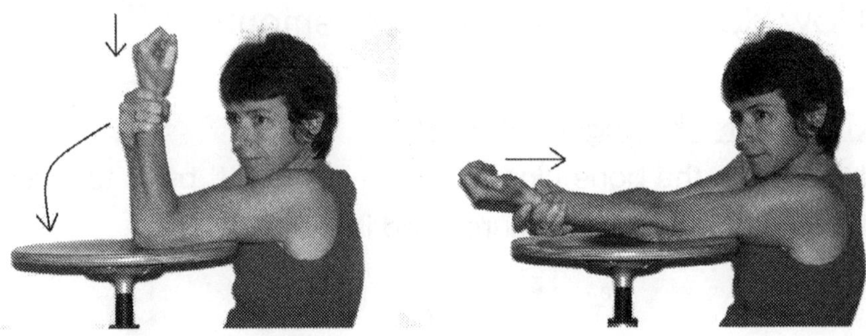

<u>2nd Thumb joint:</u>

Hold on to the phalange next to the joint, apply pressure and bring it in a half circle to the medial side of the hand.

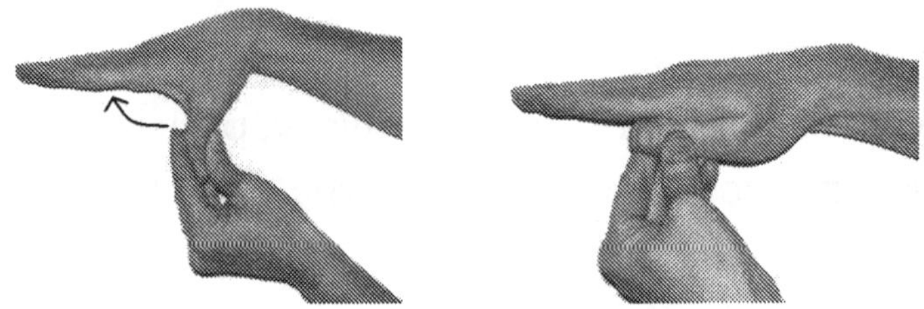

In this way you can reposition every joint and often people report amazing results in rheumatism or arthritis. It is always worth a try, you have nothing to lose and there is no risk involved.

The principle is always the same: push and bend.

3

THE DO'S AND DON'TS FOR A BETTER BACK

DO	DO NOT
• Sit straight • Get up and move around regularly • Change your sitting position • Your hip exercises regularly • Stand up correctly, always with a straight upper back • Use both sides of your body to carry if not using a backpack • Lift items using your knees • Get your weaker side to work more • Place the computer screen straight in front of yourself • Your neck exercises, especially when working in the same position the whole day • Drink enough water, best is PiMag living water (available at www.backcaresolutions.net) • Lose excess weight • Exercise on a regular basis • Use a good sleep system (see section 3.3 Additional Suggestions)	• Sit with crossed legs • Slouch your back • Sit for too long • Bend sideways to pick up anything • Carry a heavy bag on one side - use a backpack instead or change sides regularly • Underestimate your bodies signals • Lift up things using your back, use your legs instead • Wear high heels • Sleep on your tummy

3.1 The Six Master Points Of Acupressure At A Glance

Attention! Do not use acupressure during pregnancy as doing so might trigger labour.

3.1.1 Large Intestines 4

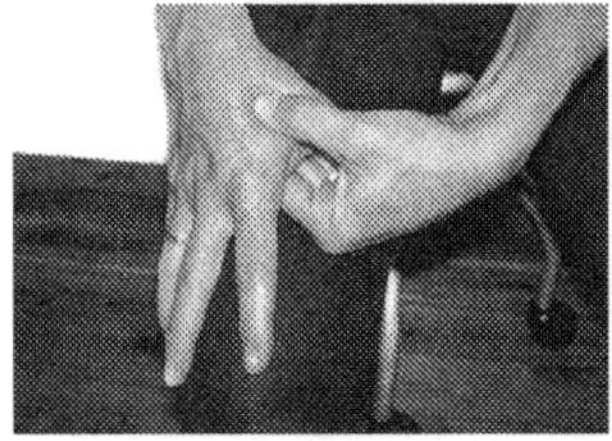

Relieves headaches and other pain, relaxes muscular tension, helps to balance the energy flow between the upper and lower parts of the body and is used to promote healthy functioning of the bowels.

This point you find in the web between your thumb and your index finger towards the end of the bony triangle.

Place your thumb on that area and your index finger underneath. Then squeeze, pressing towards the bone of the index finger.

Hold for 1 minute and repeat on the other hand. Massaging that point also helps.

3.1.2 Large Intestines 11

It is used to reduce pain in the arm, elbow and shoulder. It also can help to regulate intestinal activity.

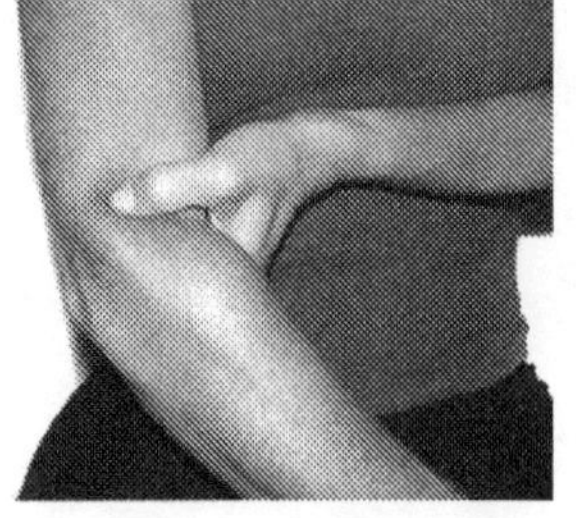

The point is positioned in the crease of your elbow.

Bring your arm into a 90° angle in front of your body and you can find the point at the lateral end of the crease on your arm close to the elbow joint.

Hold the arm close to your chest and use firm pressure with your other thumb, press for about a minute, then work on the other arm.

3.1.3 Spleen 6

This is considered the master point for healing and regulating the female organs, so it is a good point to use to regulate menstruation, ease cramps and menopause problems. It is also used together with stomach 36 (see further down) to bring vitality.

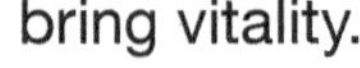

You find this point on the inside of your leg 4 finger widths above the centre of your ankle bone. It is just off the bone toward the back of your leg. Press with your index finger or thumb firmly, hold for about a minute and then release slowly. Go to the other leg

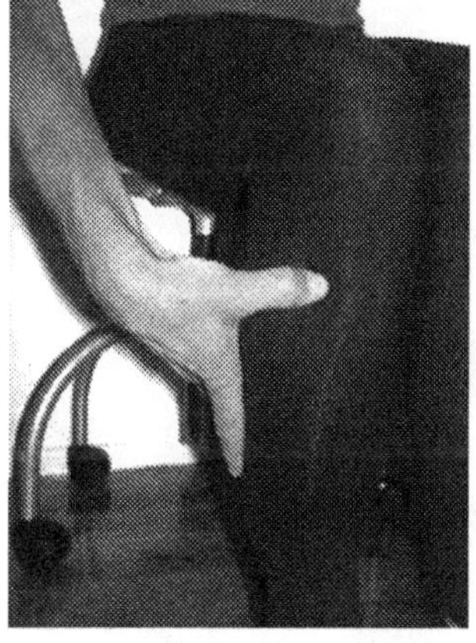

3.1.4 Stomach 36

This is the most powerful point for revitalising the whole body. By pressing this point slightly towards the knee joint you can reduce the tension in and around the knee.

This point is located 4 finger widths below the lower edge of the kneecap and one finger width laterally off the shin bone . When you have found the point, flex your foot and when you can feel the muscle move under your fingers you're right.

Hold the pressure for 1 minute and then go to the other leg.

3.1.5 Kidney 3

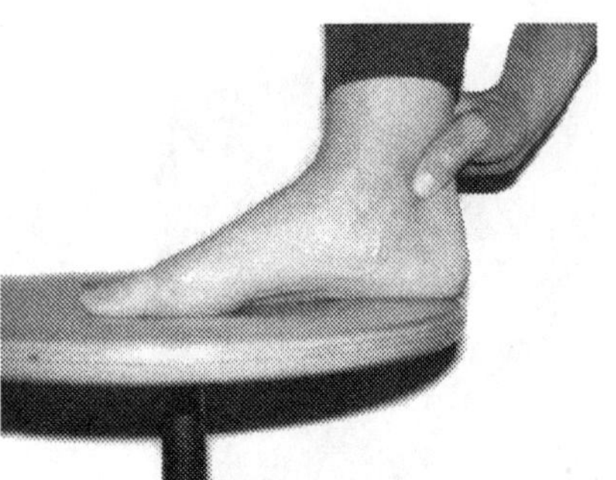

This point is considered to bring a powerful toning effect on your kidney meridian and thus on the entire body.

It is located on the inside of your ankle, halfway between the ankle bone and the Achilles tendon in the depression toward the tendon. Press with your thumb with medium to firm pressure and hold for 1 minute, then go to the other foot.

3.1.6 Gallbladder 20

This point is helpful in relieving headaches and colds, neck stiffness and pain.

To find this point place your thumbs on your earlobes, slide back towards the spine and when you hit the crease near the spine that is where you work, just under the skull.

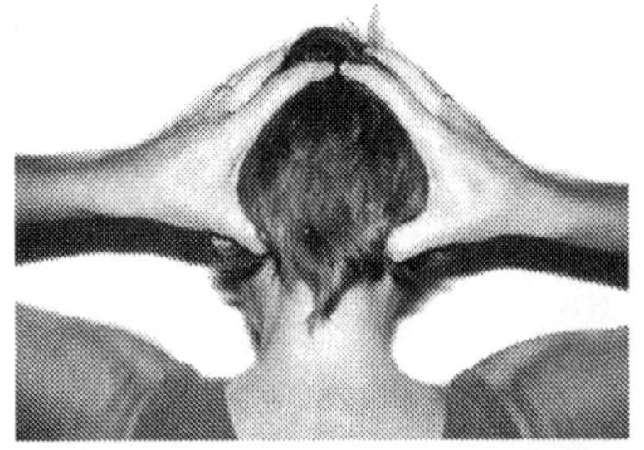

If you have difficulties finding the depression, bend your head forward and than back again. Then you will find the spot more easily.

Use medium to firm pressure and hold for at least a minute. Breathe deeply and release the pressure gradually.

3.2 Reflexology

In Reflexology you use your thumb or index finger to gently knead, rub, stroke or firmly press specific areas of the feet, the hands or the ears that are so-called reflex areas and as such relate to your entire body.

Reflexology works with the energy of life. The increased circulation through reflexology treatments removes toxins, breaks up congestion in the body and helps free up the energy lines that run through the whole body. It has been used by the Egyptians, the Indians and Incas before finding it's way into Europe and the US.

If you ask people about their experiences with reflexology you will probably most certainly get the answer, "very relaxing, soothing and energising and definitely worth a try".

To get results you should try and incorporate it into your daily routine of exercises, spend 5-10 min. on massaging your feet or hands.

Before you start your "treatment" make sure you prepare the area you want to work on. That means gently massaging your foot or hand, not on specific points but the whole area. This stimulates the area and increases blood flow.

To work on your foot or hand, rotate your ankle or your wrist in both directions To work on the reflex areas you should use your thumb as much as possible and move it slowly, applying pressure on one point after another. By doing so you create a caterpillar-like-movement with lifting and pushing down of the thumb. Never lift off completely, you should always stay in contact with the skin.

If you find it too difficult to "caterpillar" you can also use firm, slow sliding movements but still make sure you remain on the tender spots.

3.2.1 Working On Your Feet

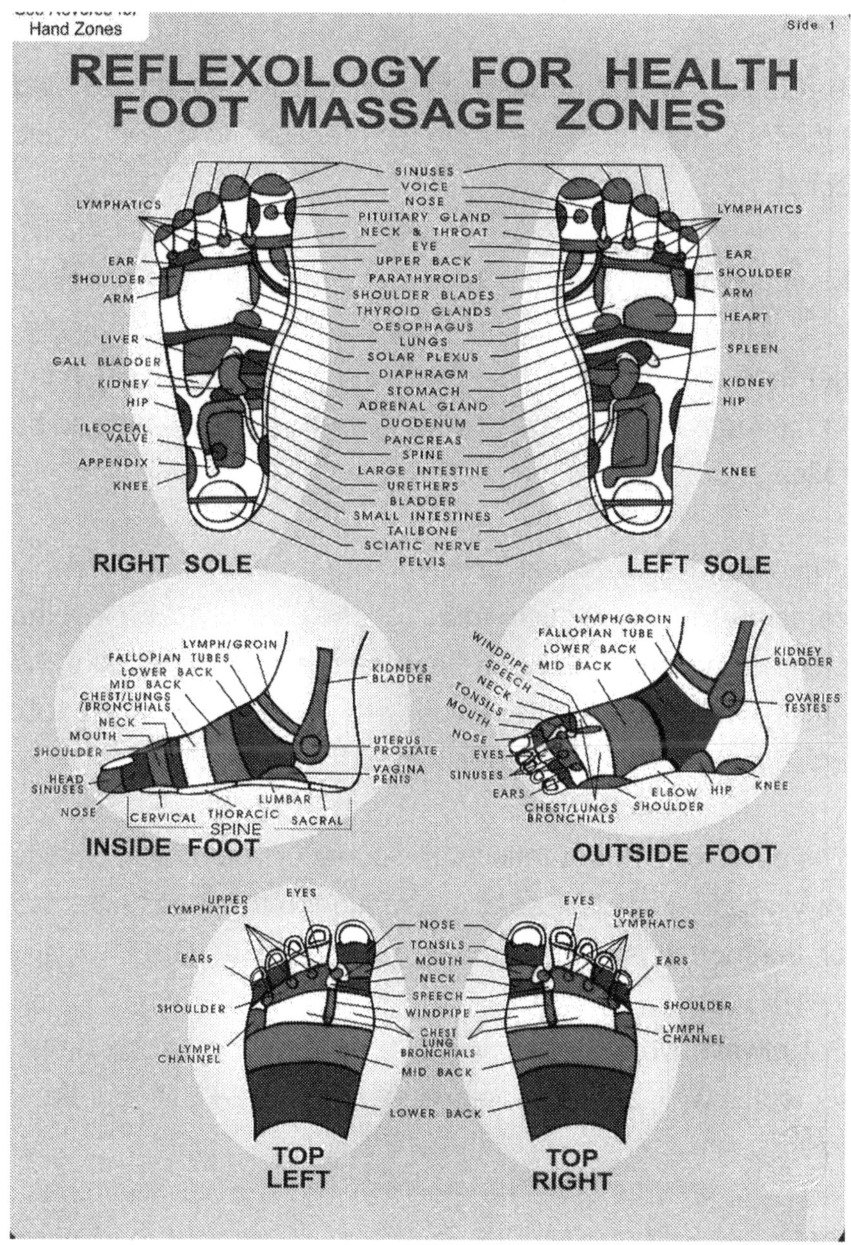

The spinal reflexes run up the inside bony edge of your feet from the big toenail bed down to the heel.

The big lump just underneath your toe represents C7 and therefore the transition from the cervical to the thoracic spine.

Most people can feel that lump just underneath their neck as well. It is not pathological for that vertebra to be slightly bigger than all the others. Use the thumb of your opposite hand to the foot you work on to slowly "caterpillar" down the spine reflex.

When you find a tender or even sore spot, rest on it, apply some pressure and micro rotate on the spot until you feel the pain easing off. When you have reached the heel, take the other way around and walk your way up towards the big toe, again resting and micro rotating on the tender or sore spots.

The curve of the foot reflects the curve of your spine. So it is very important to pay special attention to the areas reflected on the foot, where your back-problems are located.

But always work the whole spine as other parts can be affected as well, although you might not yet feel it in your back itself.

When you have worked the spine you might want to work on

the neck area as well, since a lot of tension is held in the neck and shoulders which again can cause referred back pain.

To work the neck you go to the lateral side of the big toe and walk from the top down in very little moves and apply pressure to find the tender spots. Make sure you cover the entire inside of the toe. Concentrate on tender or even sore areas, apply more pressure and micro rotate until the tension eases off. After that, place your thumb just underneath the toe joint and then using the other hand to bend the toe over the thumb you can release the tension that sits under the skull.

Hold the bent position for 15-20 seconds. Move a tiny fraction further to the side and bend again. You should do 5-6 different positions to make sure you work the whole area.

Now the shoulder girdle, a favourite for tension and tightness.

The referral area for the shoulder girdle is just underneath the toes starting at the lateral side of the big toe and ending lateral to the little toe. Work along that area in both directions, again using little moves, and remain on any tender spots to massage them even more.

For shoulder tension pay special attention to the base of the little toe and massage the whole area there, also on top of

the foot.

Useful for working on sciatic pain is the spot just on the bottom of the foot close to the heel. Squeeze with thumb and finger up the Achilles tendon.

Be careful, this can be very sensitive!

3.2.2 Working On Your Hands

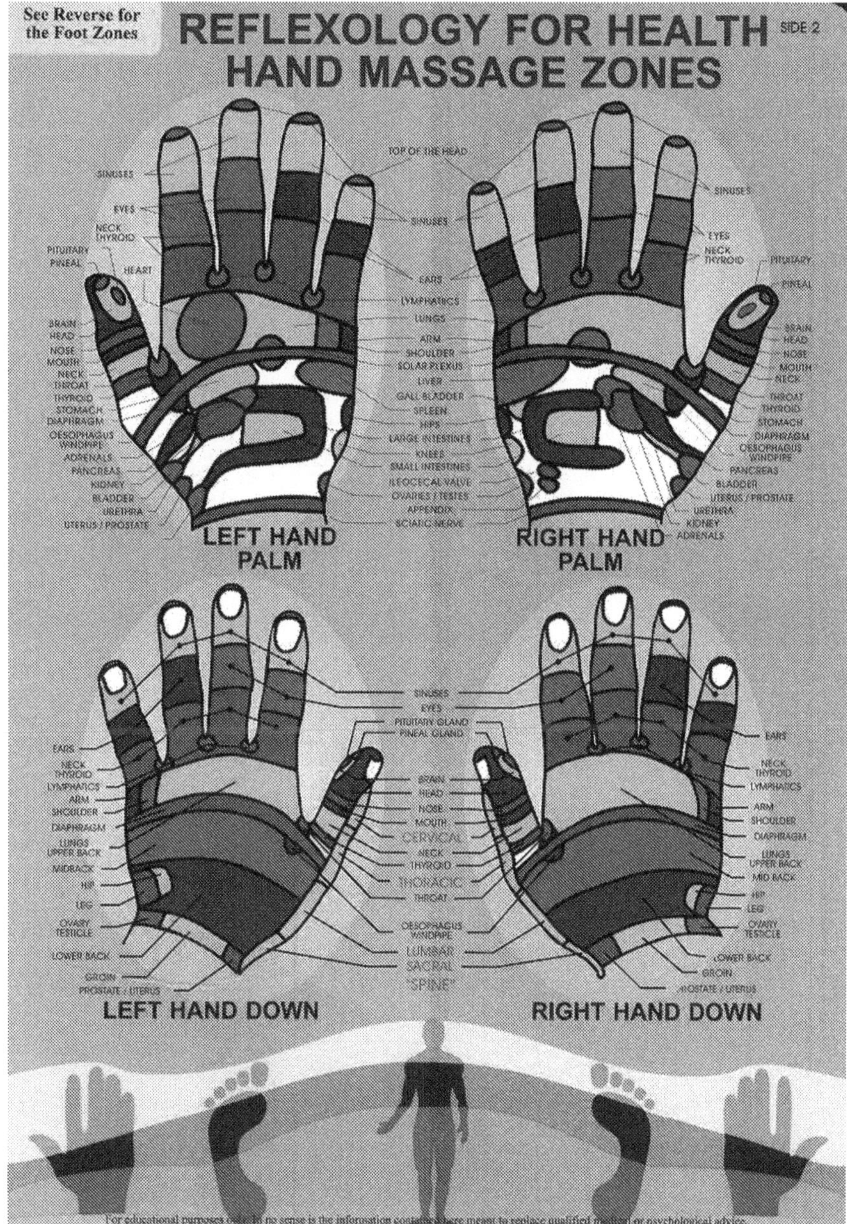

The spinal reflex area in the hands is down the medial side of the thumb along the bony edge towards the middle of the hand root.

The neck reflex is at the inside of the thumb and the skull release you can do just underneath the first joint of the thumb.

For shoulder tension you work around the base and the lowest knuckle of the little finger. The shoulder girdle is just underneath the finger bases.

For headaches it is always good to squeeze the finger tips for a few minutes. In severe headaches you might even apply pegs to each finger tip to cover as much of your head area as possible.

It looks funny but it helps - and it keeps you from working as you can't use your hands and that means you can relax for a while.

Close your eyes and feel the headache fading off.

3.3 Case studies:

If you are suffering from back pain, neck pain or headaches it might be a good idea to look out for a Dorn Spinal Therapist to get your body checked and realigned to take away the underlying causes of your pain and make your exercising more successful and beneficial for you.

To give you an idea of what other people have experienced when they decided to visit me I have listed a few case studies for you to read. Due to the Privacy Act, I cannot put in the clients's full names but if you wish to contact one of them I will try my best to arrange it for you.

When you decide you would like to see a practitioner please give me a call on ++61 2 99188057 or send me an email to barbara@backcaresolutions.net and I will give you the details of the practitioner closest to you. Thanks and enjoy reading

1. Mr. P. Nicholls, 39, Sydney

History of Condition:

Mr. Nicholls had been suffering from lower back pain for 3 years and it got consistently worse. The day he called me, he was lying on the floor and could hardly move. An X-Ray had shown no herniated or even prolapsed discs.

Findings:

Right leg slightly longer than left one, balanced in the hip joint. Right hip twisted backward, sacrum to the right, S2/L1 twisted left, T3/5 and 8 twisted left, T6 twisted right, C6 and 3 deviated to the left

Therapy:

After the first treatment Mr. Nicholls felt much better. One week went by before I saw him again, and he was now able to walk slowly and sleep through the night without any pain. He received 2 more treatments in the next 2 weeks and then we left it for 4 weeks. When I saw him again after 4 weeks he had started a light exercise routine with the home exercises. He had started to go for walks every day and started swimming which helped his back and his confidence. After 2 more treatments he was pain free and 2 years later he still is pain free.

2. Mrs. S. Aroney, 43, Sydney

History of Condition:

Headaches 2-4 times a week for the last 6 years. Only pain killers would give real relief.

Findings:

Left leg longer than right, left hip twisted, Thoracic spine deviated mainly to the right, C6 twisted left, C1 and 2 pointed to the right.

Therapy:

After 2 treatments 1 week apart, Mrs. Aroney reported no more headaches. She felt that sometimes she might get one but when she does the exercises, the sensation subsides. After 9 months she called me again for another treatment as she had one headache and didn't want to risk another one. One more treatment and I haven't seen her in 14 months now.

3. Mrs. M. Robinson, 44, Central Coast

History of Condition:

Consistent pinch in the neck, pain in her right hip down into the leg, heels hurt in both feet.

Findings:

Both legs were not correctly aligned in the joints, the right hip was considerably higher than the left and the sacrum was twisted on the right side. T5, C7 and 5 were deviated to the left.

Therapy

After 1 complete treatment the heel pain was gone completely, the hip pain had been reduced considerably and the pinch in the neck was reduced as well. When I saw her for the second treatment, her neck pain was gone as well and she only felt a slight discomfort in the right hip area. The spinal alignment had maintained very well and the most work we had to do was muscular rather than skeletal. I left it to her own decision whether or not to come for a 3rd treatment but so far she has not called in 3 months.

4. Ms. N. Balian, 17, Sydney

History of Condition:

For a few years she suffered from a consistent tightness in the neck. Her entire back felt sore and tight.

Findings:

Her left leg 2.5 cm longer than the right one and all 3 joints in that leg were affected. Also the right hip was twisted and the L4 was directing to the right side. Her entire cervical spine was pointing to the right side which explains the constant tightness. She sleeps on 2 pillows which overstretches her neck.

Therapy:

After the first complete Dorn Spinal Therapy treatments she felt much more balanced and she could virtually feel her back loosening up. Also she removed the second pillow and began to sleep only on one which contributed to a more relaxed sleep and neck as well. After one week her left leg was out of alignment again but it was easier to work on and bring back into the right position. The cervical spine stabilized and her overall feeling was much better. She kept doing her exercises and was very optimistic about her body feeling. Two weeks later she had no pain and received a Dorn check up which revealed nothing unusual. I see her for regular massages but she never complains about headaches any more.

Three weeks ago she wanted to book in for another Dorn Spinal Therapy treatment but 1 day before her appointment she called to cancel because she said that she had started again to do her exercises and the pain went after only one day.

5. Ms. N. Barsby, 44, Queensland

History of Condition:

Ms. Barsby had been suffering from a severe scoliosis since her childhood and was now at a point where she was considering surgery to stop the pain. Dorn Spinal Therapy was her last go at a treatment and I asked her to give it at least 3 treatments before she decided to go for surgery.

Findings:

Right leg 2.5 cm longer than left. Left hip considerably twisted posterior, Severe curvature in thoracic and lumbar spine, C 6 deviated to left, C1 deviated to right. Completely tightened muscles on both body sides.

Therapy:

After loosening the muscles slightly through a deep massage I started correcting her leg length and her hip. Using a special technique I worked on her skoliosis and showed her exercises she could to do at home on a daily basis. One week later we repeated the treatment and she felt confident with her home exercises.

She received regular massages in between treatments to keep the muscles as smooth as possible and after 6 weeks she came back and told me that she wasn't planning on having surgery as she felt so much better and had found a way to manage her pain. She keeps doing her exercises and comes for a check up every 4- 6 weeks.

6. H. Hunt, 5, NSW

History of Condition:

Henry complained to his mum about headaches and back pain during the night. Apparently the back pain kept him awake which also meant he did not get enough sleep and felt exhausted.

Findings:

Left leg 1 cm longer than right, Sacrum slightly twisted into coccyx as well. T2 deviated to the left, C 6 to the right and C1 to the right as well.

Therapy:

Just one gentle Dorn treatment got H. back to sleep and out of headaches and back pain. His mum called me 2 weeks later to report that he was very happy and told his friends about this weird treatment he had, where he had to swing his legs. But it did work and that is what counts. He seems to be doing his hip exercise on a regular basis.

Of course I could go on and on here but I just wanted to give you an overview of what Integrated Spinal Therapy can do for you in case the exercises on their own don't help or you have done something really bad to your back. Of course it always is important to check with your doctor in case of unusually strong pain as it could also be a herniated disc which has to be treated differently. But mostly 1-3 treatments in "normal" back problem cases can bring you back to the stage where you can manage it with the exercises. This is given that you do the exercises on a regular basis.

It is important to get your back checked before you start on your own regime of exercises as you can make things worse by not getting the original problem solved first. Exercise is always considered as prevention or maintenance but not a solution of first choice in serious problems.

3.4 Back Friendly Sports and Exercises

Yoga:

In Yoga you learn exercises that increase strength and flexibility and help prevent back problems.

If you are not sure if Yoga is good for your condition, talk to the trainer about your condition before starting your first session. They know what you can do and what you should avoid from the beginning and they will guide you in a safe way to help you build your own confidence.

Many people have excellent results with Yoga in managing their back problems. You stretch the muscles, massage the meridians and help to reduce the tension in your body. As there are now lots of yoga centres everywhere, it should not be a problem to find one close to you.

Pilates:

Pilates is a good exercise to help build up your tummy muscles and work on your posture. There are various forms of Pilates and you have to choose which one might be the most appropriate for you.

Swimming:

Swimming takes the pressure off the body and is therefore excellent as an exercise routine even if you feel too sore for other exercises. The most relaxing is backstroke, if you have an upper back problem don't do breast stroke as it is too strenuous on your upper body.

Walking:

Regular walking in good shoes and on even ground is a good exercise for your entire body. Make sure you always walk in a straight posture, with your shoulders back, chest open and head up. Your ears should be in line with your shoulders. You can use light weights in your hands to increase the benefit of the exercise and you also can strap light weights to your lower legs again to increase the benefit of the exercise. It also has been proven that regular exercise is the best medicine to prevent or lower the symptoms of menopause as well as osteoporosis.

Cross Country Skiing:

Due to the extreme stretching movement in cross country skiing this is also a fantastic exercise for your entire body. I know not everyone can take the opportunity to go cross country skiing but if you can, go for it.

3.5 Additional Suggestions

Rest:

When you experience back pain in a sudden onset, immediately lie down and rest. The best position is curled up on your side in a foetal position as this puts the least strain on your back.

If that doesn't help, lie on your back and put pillows under your knees so they are in a 90° position. This takes the pressure off the lower back. But don't rest for too long. Staying in bed for more than 2 or 3 days can make things worse as the muscles around the problem area can tense up.

Try easy movements as soon as possible and if pain persists, seek medical assistance or see a Dorn Spinal therapist (for info please send email to info@backcaresolutions.net) or another manual therapist you trust. Although often back pain can go away without any therapeutic intervention it is vital not to wait too long before you seek treatment as time in treatment can be critical. The longer you wait the longer your treatment might take.

Sleep:

Make sure you have a comfortable sleep system, consisting of a neck shaped pillow, a firm mattress and a healthy position, which is sleeping on your back. Of course it is also essential to get enough sleep and to cut down on alcohol as this brings your heart rate up thereby reducing relaxation during the night sleep.

<u>Helpful items to use in your daily life to improve your posture and your entire wellbeing:</u>

Fit ball for exercises and to sit on

Seat wedge for under your buttocks to sit straight

Traumeel homeopathic ointment to relieve symptoms of inflammation

A very good water filter system that brings you the water of life – every day!!

To see a range of all our products related to back pain and health go to www.backcaresolutions.net/products.htm

Also we have developed a home study course for those of you who want to learn Dorn Spinal Therapy in the comfort of their home. If you are interested please go to www.dorntherapycourse.com

For hands on workshops see a list of scheduled courses on www.backcaresolutions.net/workshops.htm

All the advice and tips given here do not mean you don't have to see a health practitioner ever again. They are guidelines to help you prevent pain, teach you about good posture, speed up the healing process after injuries, and maintain better health.

If you have any questions, suggestions or comments please don't hesitate to contact me on info@backcaresolutions.net

Thanks for reading and I hope you will have lots of fun and success implementing the exercises.

REFERENCES

Fleming Gerda, "Die Methode Dorn", Aurum Verlag, 1997

Godau Angelika, "Wenn Wirbel aus dem Lot greaten", Au rum Verlag, 2001

Hay Louise L., "You can heal your life", Palace Press International, 2000

Koch Andrea, Schnabel Gabriele, "Aktive Schmerzbewaeltigung bei Rueckenschmerzen", Copress Sport, 1997

Koch Helmuth, Steinhauser Hildegard, "Die Dorn-Therapie", Foitzick Verlag, 2001

Pianta, Jean-Paul, "Rueckenschmerzen muessen nicht sein", Heyne Verlag, 1997

Raslan Gamal, "Der sanfte Weg zur Mitte: Die Dorn Methode", Aurum Verlag, 2003

Reflexology chart: Ambrosia publications, 1999

Free Mystery Gift

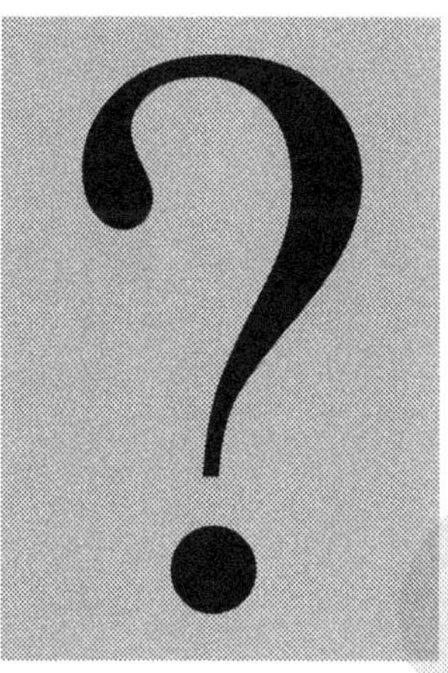

I am providing you this free mystery gift as a special thank you for purchasing my book. By reading and practicing the advice and techniques I outline in this book you are well on your way to maintaining a healthy back for life.

Free Download link:
http://www.backcaresolutions.net/freegift.htm
$30 Value

www.ingramcontent.com/pod-product-compliance
Lightning Source LLC
Chambersburg PA
CBHW031213270326
41931CB00006B/548